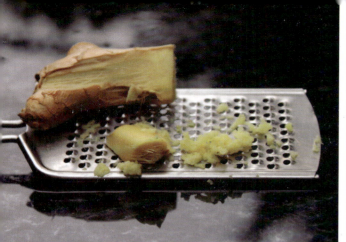
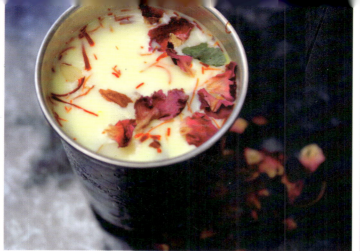
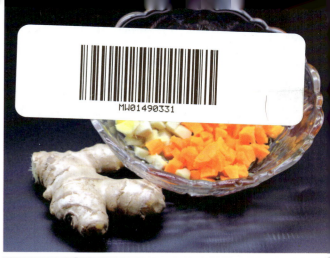

INDIAN
H ॐ ME
REMEDIES

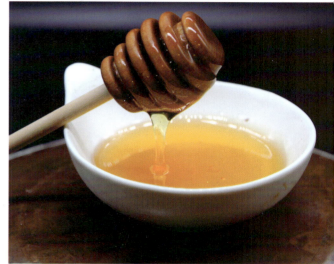
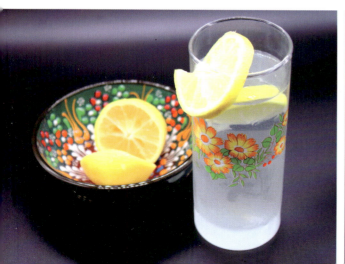
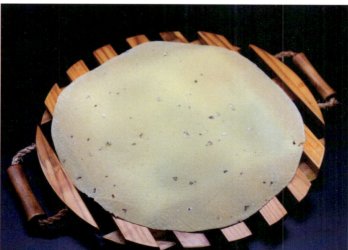
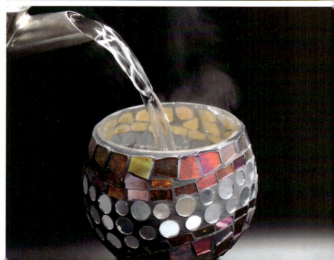

108 INDIAN HOME REMEDIES

૧૦૮ ઘરગથ્થુ ઉપચાર

Text & Photographs by Binny Sujal Nanavati

Disclaimer and a word of caution: This book is not intended as a medical reference book nor is it intended to replace the services of trained health professionals, and it should not be construed as professional medical advice. You are advised to consult with your doctor, physician or health care professional with regards to matters of your health, to discuss specific medical conditions or symptoms and in particular matter that may require diagnosis or medical attention where appropriate.

This book is a source of information and the content is intended for educational purposes only. Indian spices, herbs, and natural foods such as fruits, vegetables, grains, seeds and nuts are thought to contain medicinal, therapeutic and nourishing properties.

The author can not be held responsible for any adverse reactions to the recommendations, suggestions or remedies contained herein and the use of this book **108 Indian Home Remedies** is entirely at the reader's own discretion.

Limit of Liability/Disclaimer of Warranty: The author makes no representations or warranties with respect to the accuracy or completeness of the contents of this work and specifically disclaim all warranties, including without limitation warranties of fitness for a particular purpose. No warranty may be created or extended by sales or promotional materials, The advice and strategies contained herein may not be suitable for every situation. This work is sold with the understanding that if medical professional assistance is required, the services of a competent medical professional person should be sought. The author shall not be held liable for damages arising here from, including but not limited to special, consequential or incidental damages. The fact that an individual, organization, or website is referred to in this work as a citation and/or potential source of further information does not mean that the author endorses the information the individual, organization, or website may provide or recommendations they/it may make. Further, readers should be aware that websites listed in this work may have changed or disappeared between when this work was written and when it is read.

ISBN: 978-1-7346981-0-7 (hardcover)
The Library of Congress Cataloging-in-Publication Data is available upon request.

Binnys LLC, Texas, USA
E-mail: binnynanavati@gmail.com
Website: www.binnynanavati.com

Bharat Graphics, A-212, Sumel-9, Nr. Maheshwari Estate, Dhudheswar Road, Shahibaug - 380 004 Gujarat, India
E-mail: bharatgraphics1@gmail.com

Printed in India

First Edition, July 2020
10 9 8 7 6 5 4 3 2 1

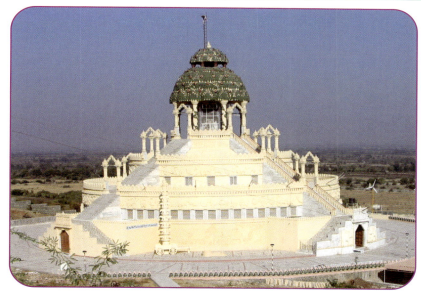

Parmātmānī Krupāthī anē Pappā-Mummy nā Aśīrvādthī

પરમાત્માની કૃપાથી અને પપ્પા મમ્મીના આશીર્વાદથી

With God's grace and blessings from my Mom & Dad and my Mother-in-Law & Father-in-Law.

*This book is dedicated to my **Sujal**,
and our right hand & left hand, **Sunay & Saavan.***

*I **Love** you all!*
Binny

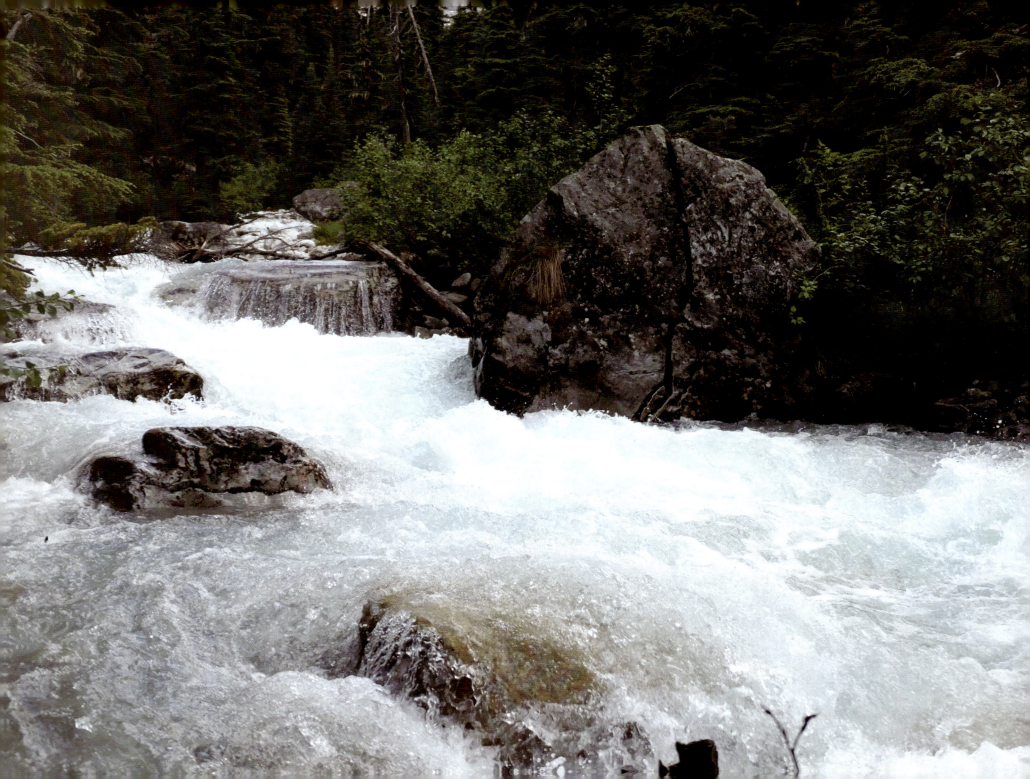

CONTENTS

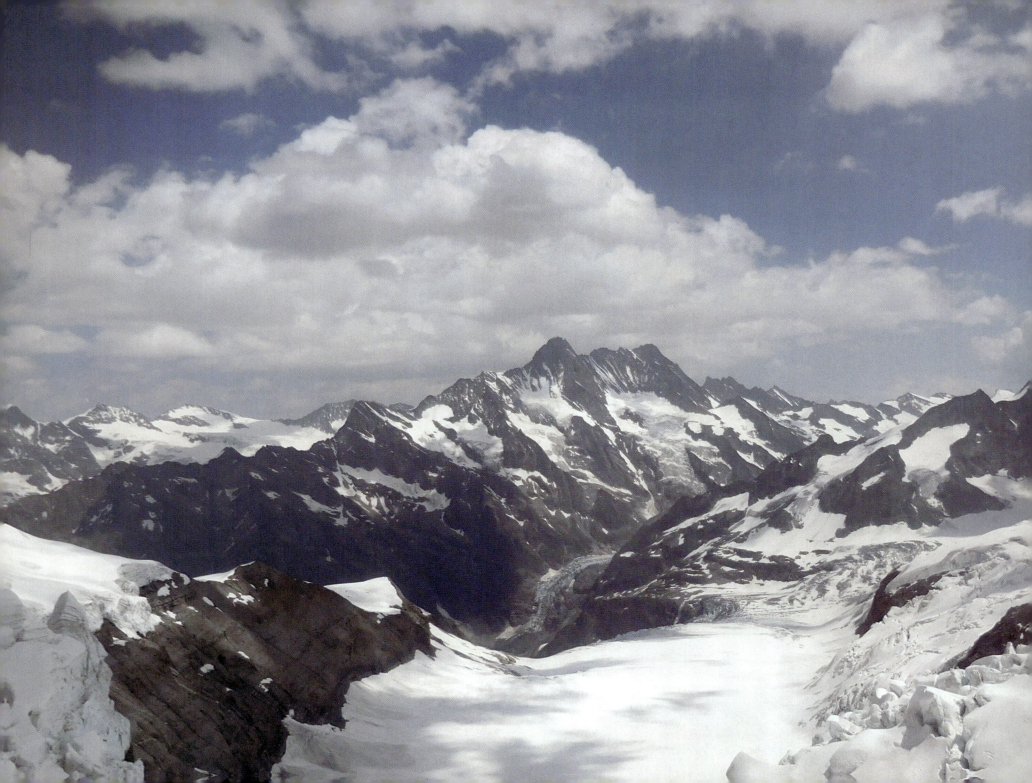

Listing of Conditions

*"The most important principle of environment is that
you are not the only element."*
—Mahāvīra Bhaghwān (599 BCE – 527 BCE)
*24th and last Tirthankara ("Ford-maker", spiritual pioneer and teacher) of the Jain Dharma (righteous path)
spiritual successor of the 23rd Tirthankara Parśhvanathā Bhaghwān*

Remedy Lookup

"The greatest distance between two people is misunderstanding."
—Anonymous

Condition	Remedy Name	In English	Page
Acidity	1. Chokhani Faki	1. Anti-Acidity Rice Treatment	21
Acne	2. Multani Mati	2. Fuller's Earth Healing Clay Mask	23
	3. Besan ane Doodh	3. Gram Flour Milk Face Mask	25
Allergies	4. Deevel	4. Castor Oil Drop	27
Anxiety	5. Haldar Mithanu Doodh	5. Turmeric Latte	29
Arthritis	6. Nilgiri Malish	6. Eucalyptus Oil Massage	31
Asthma	7. Aakhi Harde	7. Therapeutic Dry Fruit	33
Brain Development	8. Badam	8. Brain Tonic Almonds with Metabolism Booster	35
Breath Freshener	9. Variyalino Mukhvas	9. Flavorful Delicious Fennel	37
Canker Sores	10. Momathi Lalpadvi	10. Salt Water Solution	39
Chapped Lips	11. Ghee Hothh Mate	11. Lip Massage	41
Cholesterol	12. Aadunu Pani	12. Ginger Coolant Juice	43
Cold	13. Aaduno Rus	13. Ginger Detox Juice	45
	14. Soonth Pipramulni Goli	14. Ginger Donut Balls	47
	15. Garam Pani Pivanu	15. Hot Water Sips	49
Colic	16. Hing Chopadvanu	16. Asafoetida Tummy Paste	51
Congestion	17. Elaichi ane Madh	17. Cardamom Honey Nectar	53
	18. Amba Haldarno Tukado	18. Mango Ginger Gum	55
Constipation	19. Haldar Limbunu Pani	19. Turmeric Detox	57
	20. Anjeer	20. Fiber Rich 'n Regular Figs	59
Cough	21. Elaichina Fotra	21. Roasted Cardamom Pod Syrup	61
	22. Madh ane Limbu	22. Honey Lemon Drop	63
	23. Rainu Pani	23. Mustard Seeds Drink	65
	24. Madh ane Haldar	24. Turmeric Honey Elixir	67
	25. Soonthni Ladudi	25. Immune Boosting Balls	69
	26. Shekelu Laving	26. Roasted Clove Drops	71
	27. Laving ane Madh	27. Clove Infused Honey	73

Condition	Remedy Name	In English	Page
Cough	28. Dalia	28. High Protein Roasted Chana	75
	29. Kacho Papad	29. Unroasted Raw Papadum	77
Dark Circle	30. Ankho Mate Gheenu Malish	30. Ghee Eye Massage	79
	31. Kesarnu Malish	31. Saffron Eye Mask	81
Dehydration	32. Limbunu Sharbat	32. Thirst Quencher Lemonade	83
Detox	33. Upvas	33. Self-Discipline 1-Day Water Fast	85
	34. Chhath	34. Power Pack 2-Days Water Fast	87
	35. Attham	35. Transformational 3-Days Water Fast	89
	36. Ayambil	36. Forever Cleanse for Victory over Taste	91
Diabetes	37. Karelano Rus	37. Reverse Diabetes Smoothie	93
	38. Hardenu Pani	38. Diabetes Dried Superfruit	95
Diarrhea	39. Lassi	39. Relaxing Yogurt Beverage	97
	40. Dahi ane Bhaat	40. Comfort Curd Rice	99
	41. Khadi Saakar	41. Rock Sugar Drink	101
	42. Kali Cha | Kophee	42. Black Tea or Coffee	103
	43. Kacha Kela	43. Unripe Green Banana	105
Digestion	44. Gheenu Pani	44. Gut Soother	107
	45. Uliyu	45. Tongue Scraper	109
	46. Pani	46. Plain Water	111
	47. Fotrawali Dalni Khichadi	47. Moong Dal Khichadi	113
	48. Tambano Loto	48. Water from Copper Vessel	115
Dry Nose	49. Nas	49. Soothing Steam Facial Inhaler	117
Dry Skin	50. Besan ane Dahi	50. Gram Flour Curd Face Mask	119
Ear Infection	51. Garam Shek	51. Warm Compress	121
Energy Boost	52. Kelu	52. Energy Booster Banana	123
Eye Disease	53. Kesar nu Shrikhand	53. Saffron-Infused Yogurt	125
Fatigue	54. Masala Cha	54. Aromatic Chai Gujarati Style	127

Condition	Remedy Name	In English	Page
Fatigue	55. Thandai	55. Aromatic Spiced Frappe Milkshake	129
	56. Aadu Fudinano Ukalo	56. Ginger Mint Shot	131
Fever	57. Kansani Vadki	57. Ayurvedic Foot Massage	133
	58. Mithana Panina Pota	58. Salt Water Sponge	135
	59. Ukalo	59. Spiced Shot	137
	60. Bajrino Kadho	60. Creamy Millet Porridge	139
Flu	61. Ganthodano Ukalo	61. Zesty Peepramul Shot	141
Gas	62. Hing Marino Ukalo	62. Asafoetida Pepper Shot	143
	63. Methi	63. Soaked Fenugreek	145
Good Health Newborn	64. Ghasaro	64. Health Tonic	147
Gum Disease	65. Haldar Chopadvi	65. Turmeric Gum Massage	149
Hair Fall	66. Vaal Mate Tel Malish	66. Nourishing Hair Massage	151
Headache	67. Chandan Lagavo	67. Sandalwood Creamy Gel Paste	153
Heart Disease	68. Akhrot	68. Anti-Oxidant Rich Walnuts	155
Immunity Boost	69. Badam Pistanu Doodh	69. Spiced Almond Latte	157
	70. Golnu Pani	70. Blissful Jaggery Drink	159
	71. Lavingnu Pani	71. Soothing Clove Tea	161
	72. Gundarni Raab	72. Edible Gum Almond Porridge	163
Indigestion	73. KhasKhas	73. Poppy Seeds Ghee Syrup	165
Insomnia	74. Jaiphalnu Doodh	74. Sleepy Nutmeg Elixir	167
Irritable Bowel Syndrome	75. Jeeravali Chhas	75. Cumin Spiced Buttermilk	169
Joint Pain	76. Soonth Pipramulnu Doodh	76. Ginger Peepramul Latte	171
Lower Blood Pressure	77. Kali Draksh	77. Tasty Soaked Black Raisins	173
Metabolism	78. Amlanu Pani	78. Natural Fat Burner Tea	175
	79. Alsi ane Dahi	79. Powerhouse Flaxseeds with Curd	177
	80. Trifalanu Pani	80. Triphala Tea Infusion	179
Motion Sickness	81. Laving Chavavu	81. Relaxing Clove Gum	181

Condition	Remedy Name	In English	Page
Mucus	82. Madh ane Mari	82. Honey 'n Pepper Detox Tea	183
Muscle Ache	83. Tel Malish	83. Sesame Oil Ayurvedic Massage	185
Nausea	84. Jeeranu Pani	84. Cumin Infused Tea	187
Nose Bleed	85. Ghee Naak Mate	85. Ghee Nose Ointment	189
Plague	86. Trifalana Kogla	86. Triphala Mouth Wash	191
Poor Vision	87. Dooti Upar Malish	87. Therapeutic Belly Button Massage	193
Protein Boost	88. Moongnu Pani	88. Moong Detox Soup	195
	89. Tuver Dalni Khichadi	89. Rice and Lentil Super Food	197
Rash	90. Deevel Malish	90. Castor Oil Lotion	199
Regular Bowel Movement	91. Navsheku Pani	91. Lukewarm Water Routine	201
Rejuvenation	92. Saakarnu Pani	92. Refreshing Sweet Water	203
Runny Nose	93. Madh ane Aadu	93. Honey Ginger Solution	205
Sinus	94. Ajmanu Pani	94. Ajwain Water	207
	95. Aadu Limbuno Rus	95. Soothing Lemon Ginger Tea	209
Sore Muscles	96. Kesar Pistanu Doodh	96. Aromatic Saffron Latte	211
Sore Throat	97. Kala Mari	97. Peppery Toffee Lozenge	213
	98. Haldarnu Pani	98. Golden Turmeric Water	215
	99. Mithana Panina Kogla	99. Salt Water Gargle	217
Split Ends	100. Vaalma Ghee Lagavo	100. Ghee Hair Mask	219
Stomach Ache	101. Methini Chhas	101. Fenugreek Spiced Buttermilk	221
	102. Ajmani Faki	102. Ajwain Syrup	223
	103. Elaichi Ghee	103. Cardamom Peepramul Syrup	225
Stye	104. Kesar	104. Anti-Inflammatory Saffron Healing Paste	227
Weight Loss	105. Methina Dana	105. Weight Loss Fenugreek Drink	229
	106. Limbu ane Fudinanu Pani	106. Lemon-Infused Refresher	231
Wheezing	107. Ajmano Shek	107. Carom Seeds Thermal Hot Pack	233
Wound	108. Haldar Lagavavi	108. Turmeric Topical Paste	235

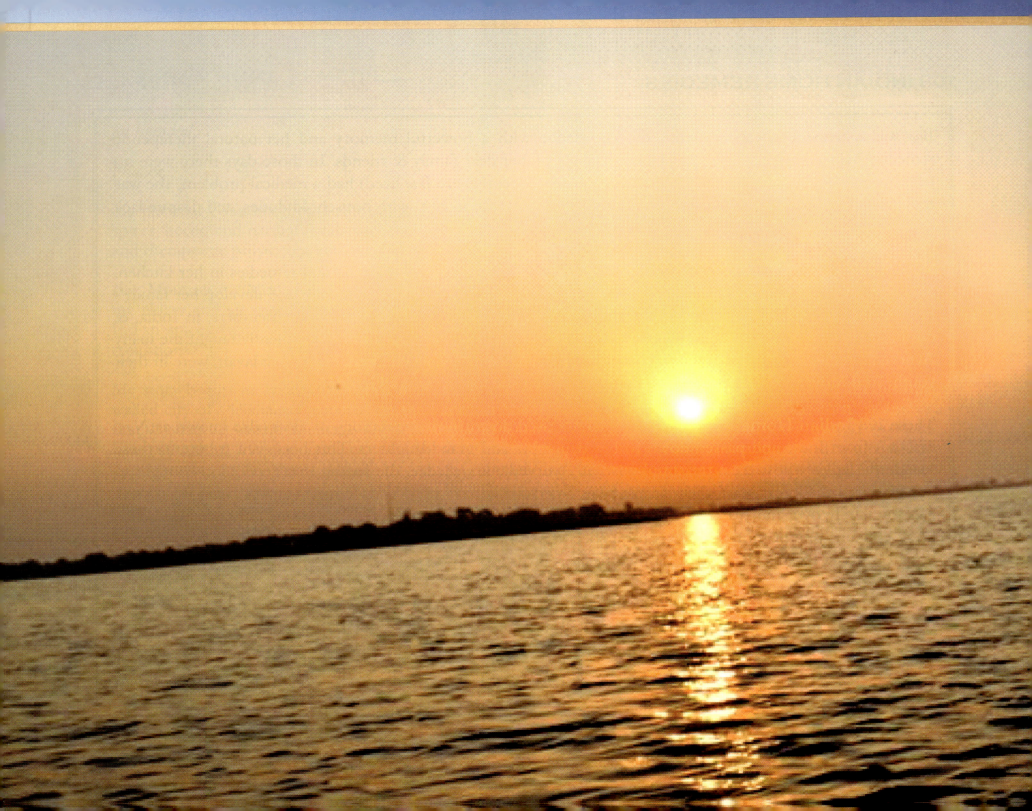

108 Indian Home Remedies

*"Be faithful in small things because
it is in them that your strength lies."*
—Mother Theresa

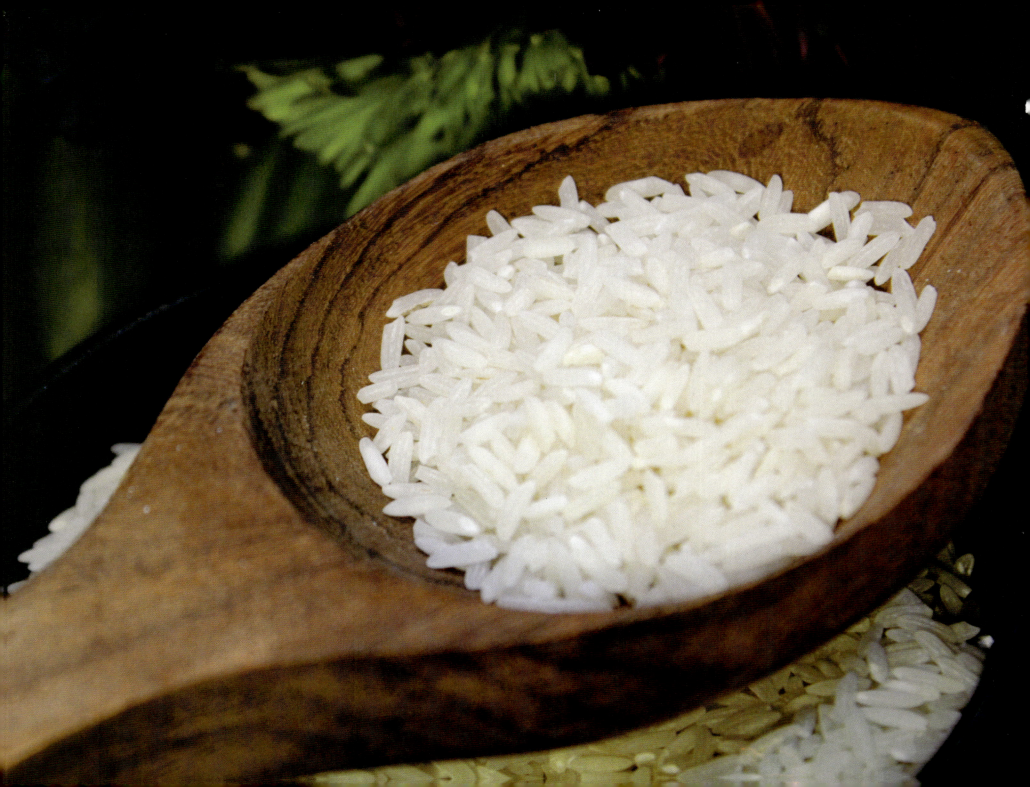

1. Chōkhānī Fākī (Anti-Acidity Rice Treatment)
ચોખાની ફાકી

LOWERS ACID REFLUX AND ACIDITY APPROXIMATELY 15 MINUTES AFTER APPLICATION

- Take 8-10 **UNCOOKED RAW RICE GRAINS**

- Put rice grains in your mouth (without chewing) and immediately swallow with a full 8 ounce glass of **LUKEWARM WATER**

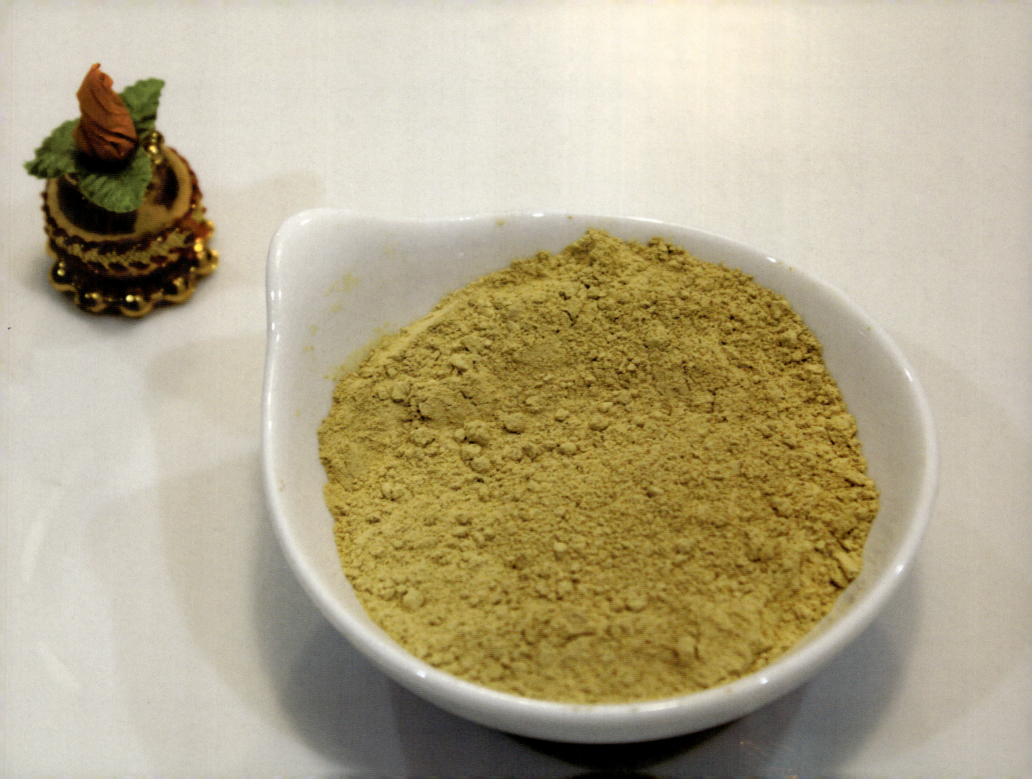

2. Multānī Māṭī (Fuller's Earth Healing Clay Mask)
મુલતાની માટી

REDUCE PORES, ACNE AND FOR SMOOTH, CLEAR & GLOWING SKIN

- Wash your hands
- Take 2 teaspoons of **FULLER'S EARTH** in a small bowl
- Add 1 teaspoon of **ORGANIC ROSE WATER**
- Mix to get a smooth paste (add more rose water if any lumps)
- Apply this smooth cooling face mask paste as an even layer on your face (forehead, under eyes, cheeks, on top of nose, below nose, under chin)
- Leave it on your skin for <u>15 minutes</u>
- Rinse with water
- Repeat twice a week as needed

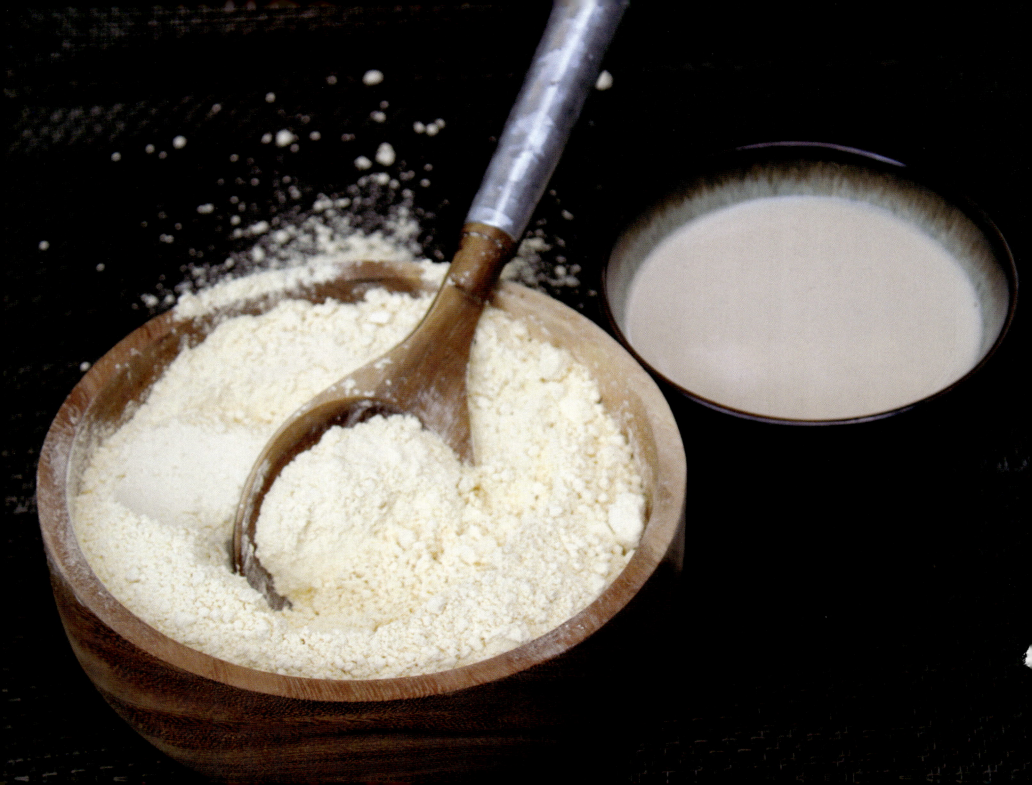

3. Bēsan anē Doodh (Gram Flour Milk Face Mask)

બેસન અને દૂધ

IMPROVE ACNE, UNCLOGS PORES, BRIGHTENS COMPLEXION

- Take 3 tablespoons of **GRAM FLOUR** in a small bowl

- Pour 5 tablespoons of **MILK** of your choice in the bowl and mix to create thick paste (add more flour/milk to get it to right consistency)

- Apply this thick face mask paste as an even layer on your face (under eyes, forehead, cheeks, on top of nose, below nose, under chin)

- Leave it on your skin for 15 minutes to <u>dry naturally</u>

- Rinse with water

- Pat your skin dry

- Repeat every 4 days as needed

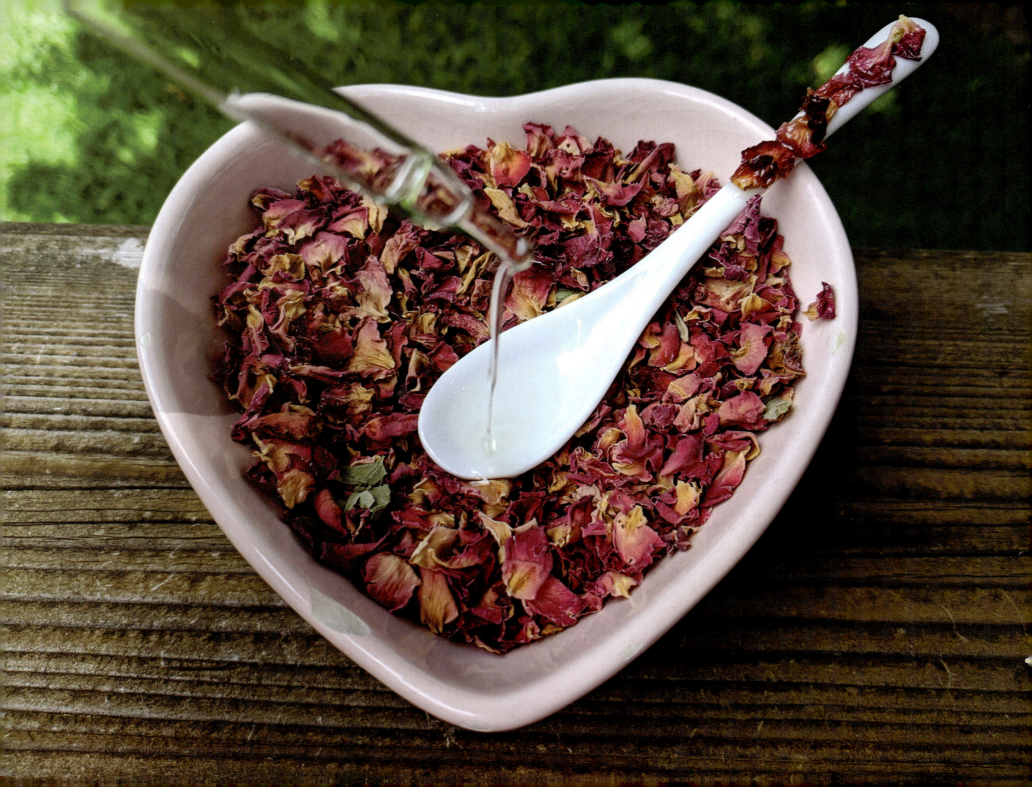

4. Deevēl (Castor Oil Drop)
દીવેલ

FOR COLD, SINUS PRESSURE, SEASONAL ALLERGIES

- Tilt your head backwards in a comfortable position (standing, sitting, lying down)

- Place a drop of **CASTOR OIL** in each nostril via a dropper or a clean finger to gently lubricate the nasal passage

- Breathe deeply to allow oil to penetrate internal nasal passages

- Repeat for <u>both nostrils total 3x in each sitting</u>

- Massage external nasal area for a few minutes

- Follow above process in the morning or before going to bed

- Repeat as needed

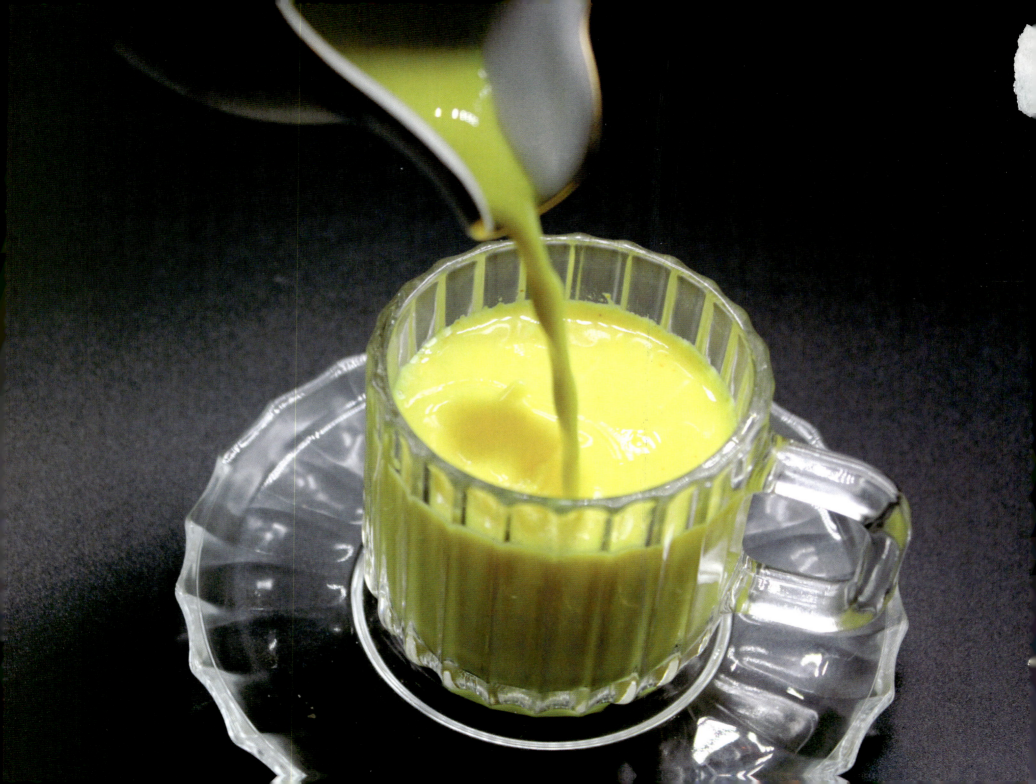

5. Haḷdar Mīthānu Doodh (Turmeric Latte)
હળદર મીઠાનું દૂધ

BENEFICIAL FOR ANXIETY, SLEEP, CONGESTION, COLDS, CLEARS MUCUS IN THE THROAT

- Heat 1 teaspoon of **PURE ORGANIC GHEE** in a small saucepan over medium heat
- Add ½ teaspoon **GROUND ORGANIC TURMERIC POWDER**
- Immediately add 1 cup of **MILK** of your choice (optional: replace 1 cup of milk with 1 cup of **WATER**)
- Stir <u>continuously</u>
- Reduce heat to medium-low and let it cook until the flavors blend
- Turn off heat when it comes to boil
- Add ¼ teaspoon **SALT** (adjust quantity as per your taste) and mix well
- Pour into a mug and enjoy this wonderful drink of wellness while hot
- Repeat 2 times a day as needed

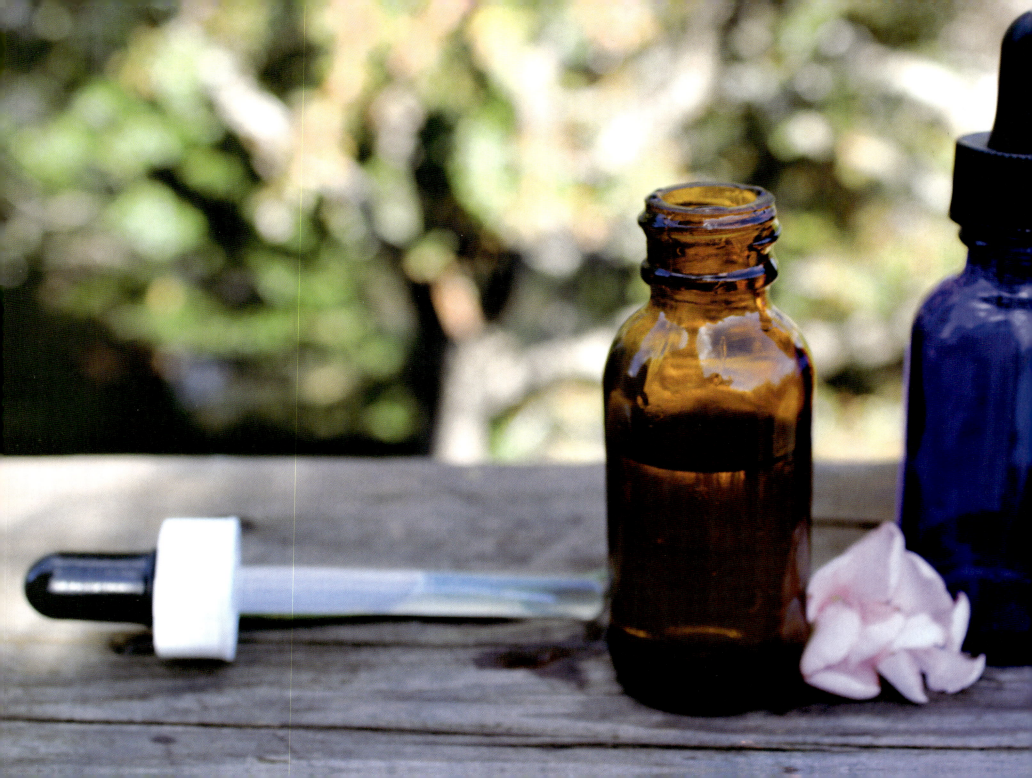

6. Nīlgirī Māliśh (Eucalyptus Oil Massage)
નીલગિરી માલિશ

FOR RELIEF FROM JOINT PAIN AND ARTHRITIS

- Wash your hands

- Topically apply 2 drops of **EUCALYPTUS OIL** to affected area of pain

- Rub in <u>circular motion</u> for 5-7 minutes

- Wash hands thoroughly afterward

- Repeat daily as needed

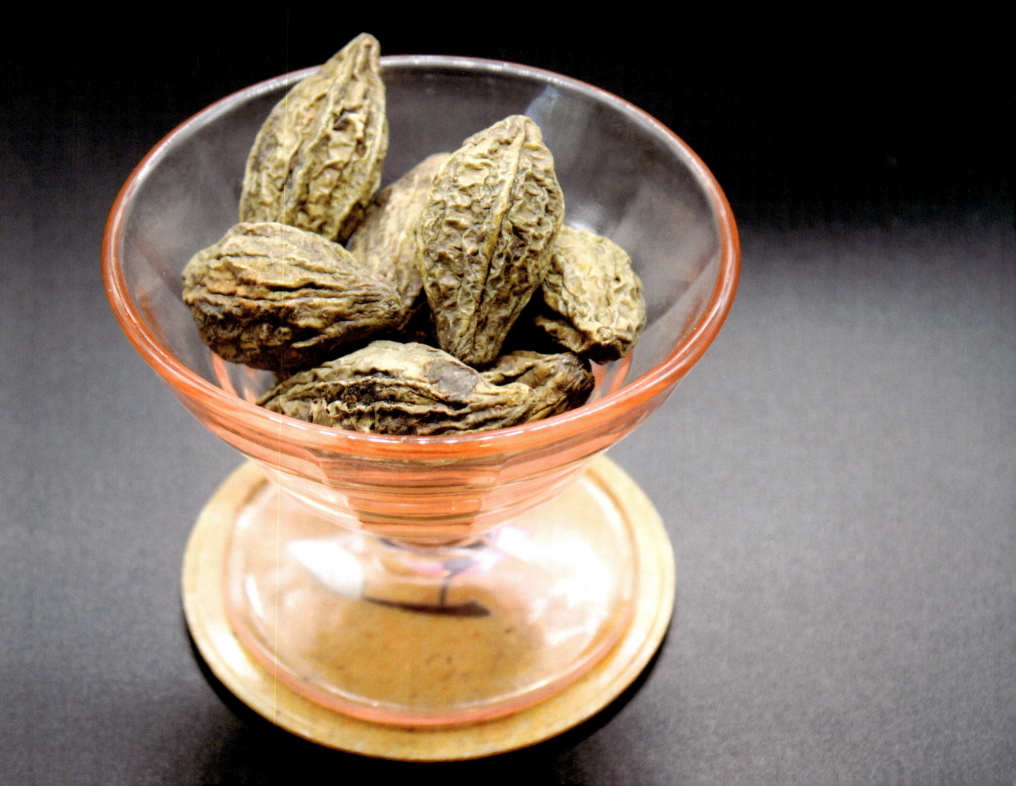

7. Āakhī Harḍē (Therapeutic Dry Fruit)
આખી હરડે

FOR NAGGING COUGH AND ASTHMA IN BABIES

- Wash your hands
- Wash flat grinding stone with **HOT WATER** and let it dry
- Rub one **HARDE** (also known as **HARITAKI**) on the grinding stone for 4 full strokes
- Use your fingers to collect what is left on the stone to a clean, sterile spoon
- Mix with ⅛ teaspoon **ORGANIC HONEY** using your finger
- Immediately give this tonic to the baby to swallow (total ¼ teaspoon in volume; increase dosage to ½ teaspoon after 3 years in age)
- Wash harde dry fruit with water and <u>dry after use</u>. Store in an airtight container for future use
- Repeat daily as needed

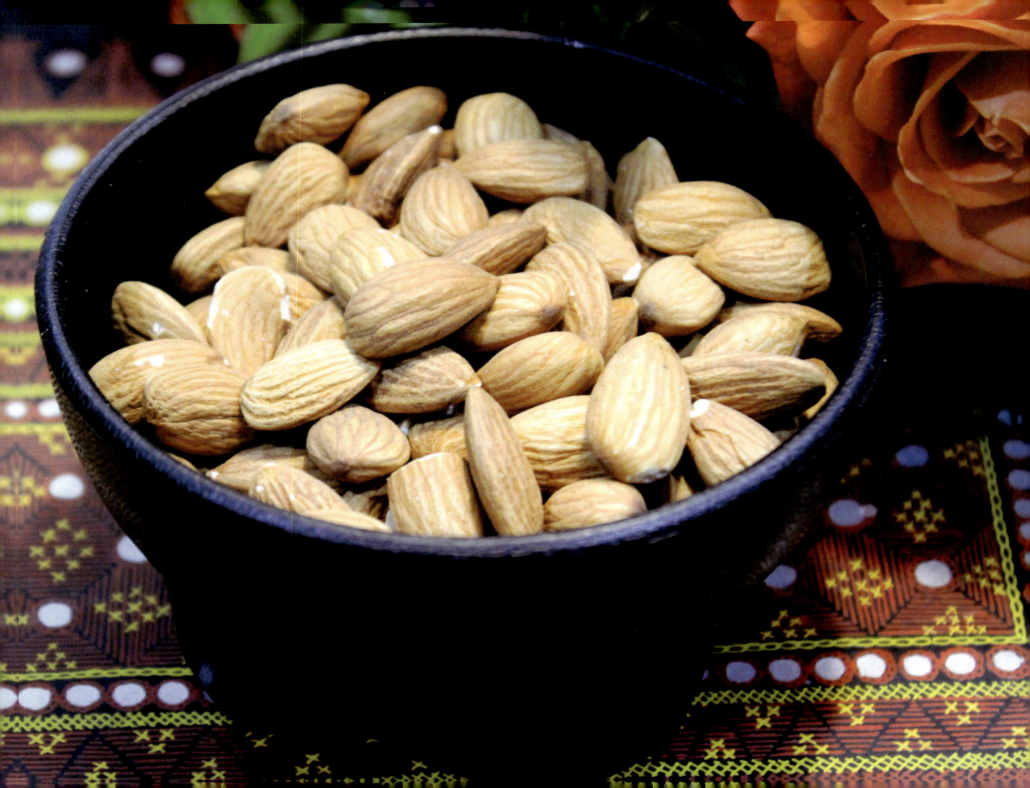

8. Badām (Brain Tonic Almonds with Metabolism Booster)

બદામ

IMPROVES BRAIN POWER AND PROMOTES WEIGHT LOSS

- Soak 7 **RAW ORGANIC WHOLE ALMONDS** in a ¼ cup of **WATER** overnight at room temperature

- Cover the bowl with a lid

- In the morning drain the water and rinse the nuts

- Remove the <u>outer peel</u>

- Chew peeled almonds slowly until it becomes liquid and swallow

- Repeat daily

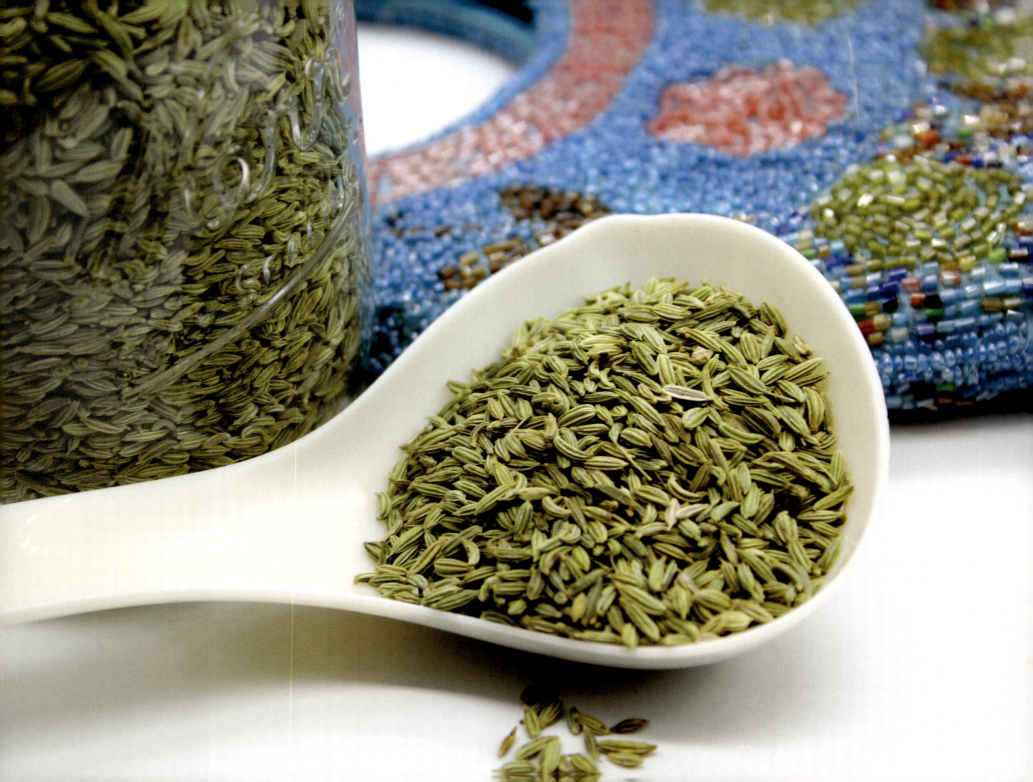

9. Variyāḷīnō Mukhvās (Flavorful Delicious Fennel)
વરિયાળીનો મુખવાસ

BREATH FRESHENER, AIDS DIGESTION

- Roast ½ cup **FENNEL SEEDS** in a pan over low heat for 2 minutes stirring regularly with a spatula

- When fennel seeds cool down, keep in an airtight container

- Put ½ teaspoon roasted fennel seeds in a spoon

- <u>Slowly chew</u> and swallow 1-2 teaspoons of fennel seeds after a meal

- Optional: open 4 green **CARDAMOM PODS**. Mix black curshed seeds from the pod, 4-6 teaspoons of **ROCK SUGAR**, ¼ cup of roasted fennel seeds and ¼ cup of **FLAXSEEDS**. Keep in an airtight container. Take 1-2 teaspoons of this mixture, slowly chew and swallow

- Avoid drinking water for 30 minutes afterward

- Repeat daily after each meal

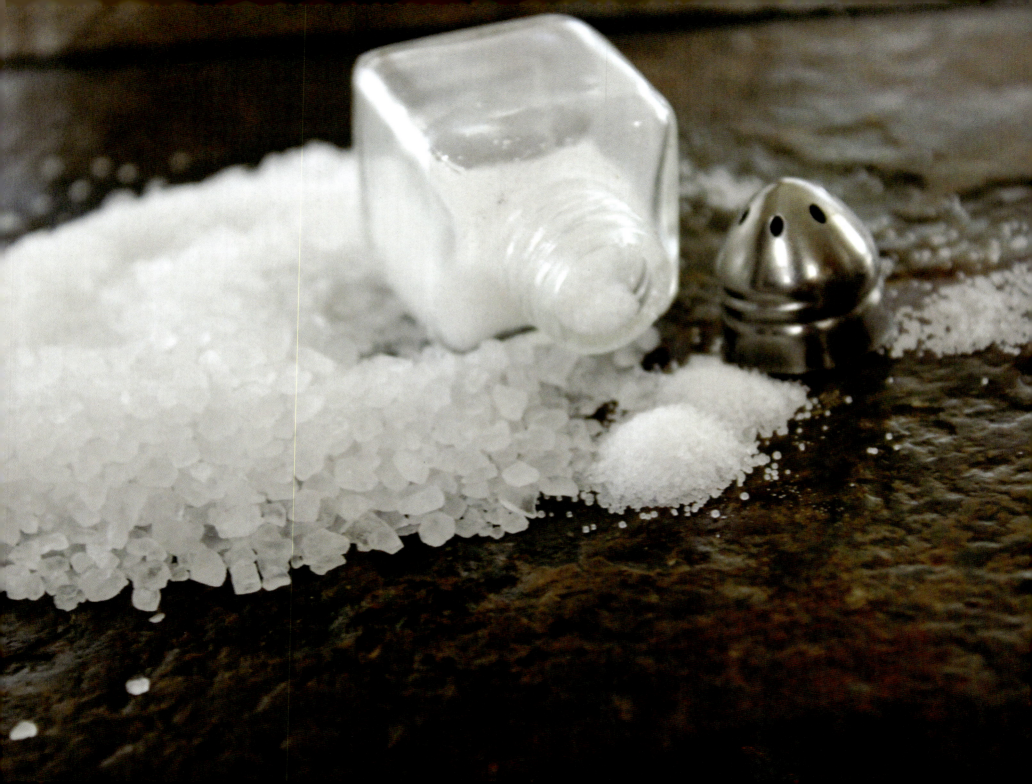

10. Mōmāthī Lāḷpāḍvī (Salt Water Solution)
મોમાંથી લાળપાડવી

TO REDUCE CANKER SORE IN THE MOUTH

- Topically apply ½ teaspoon of **SALT** <u>directly on the sore</u>

- Lean over sink and allow the water that discharges from the mouth to ooze out

- After a minute rinse mouth with mixture of 1 teaspoon of salt and 1 cup of warm **WATER**

- Repeat 2 times a day for relief

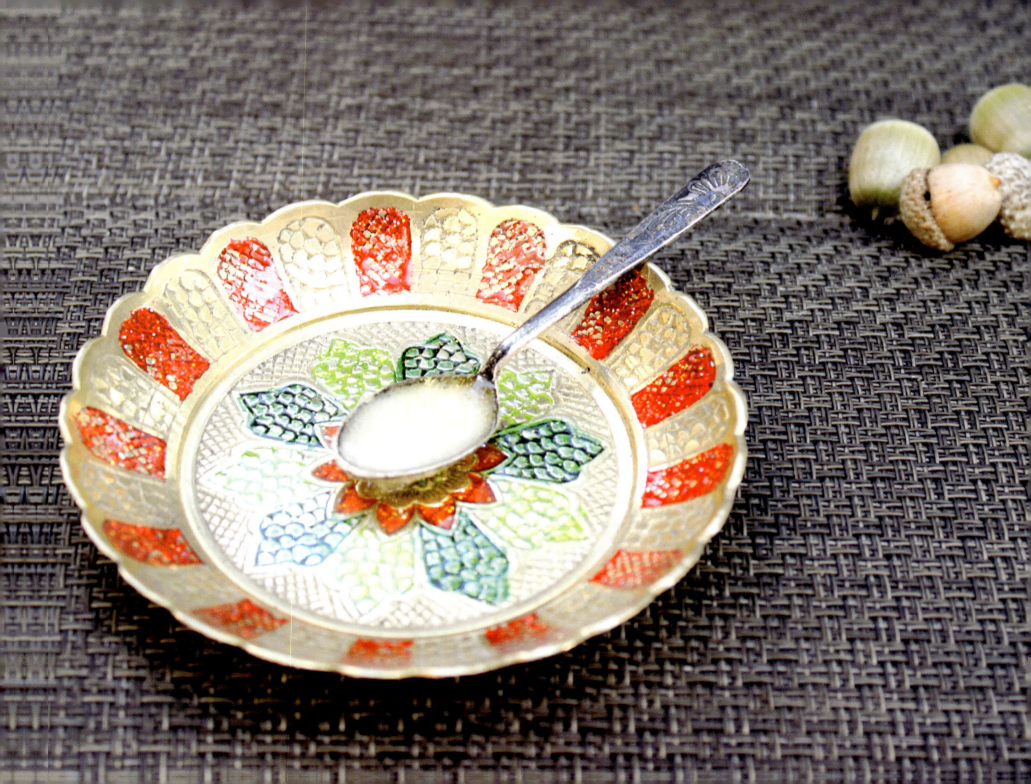

11. Ghee Hōthh Mātē (Lip Massage)

ઘી હોઠ માટે

HELP SOFTEN CHAPPED LIPS AND A MOISTURIZER

- Wash your hands

- Before going to bed, take 1 drop of **PURE ORGANIC GHEE** on your fingertip and apply over your lips

- Massage the area <u>gently</u>

- Leave it overnight

- Rinse with water in the morning

- Repeat daily as needed

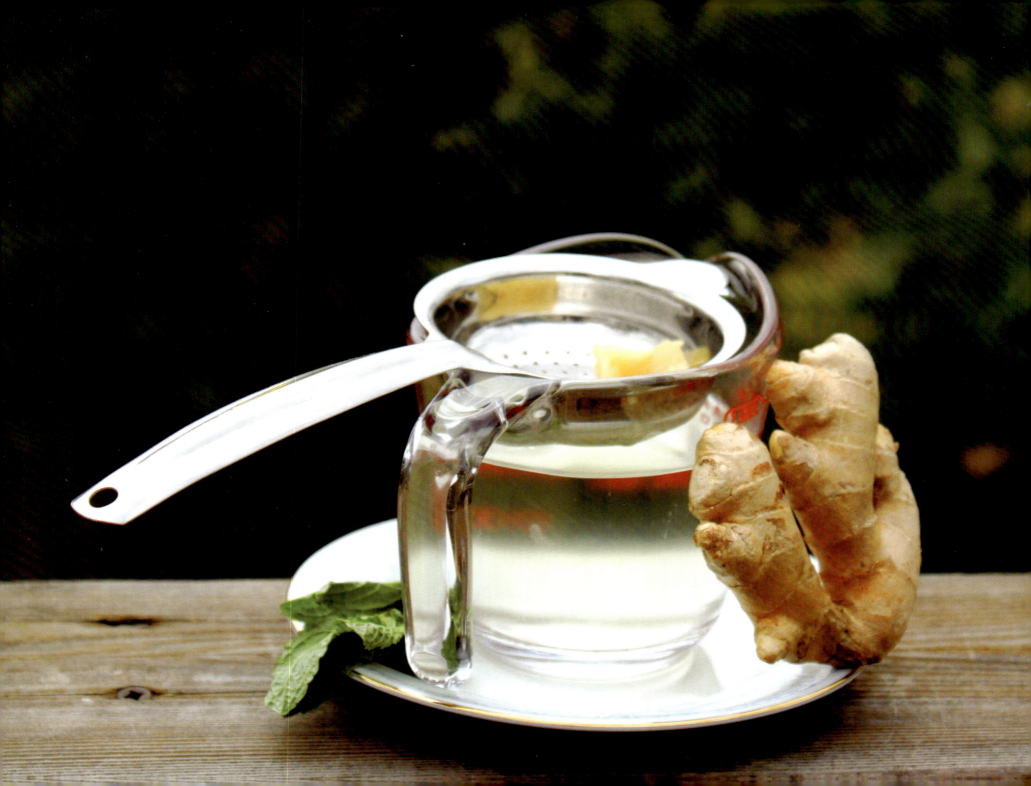

12. Āadunu Pāṇī (Ginger Coolant Juice)

આદુનું પાણી

LOWER CHOLESTEROL, SOOTHES THROAT DURING COUGH, COLD, SINUS OR CONGESTION

- Peel 2-inch fresh **GINGER**
- Cut into ¼ inch pieces and crush
- Put 1 cup of **WATER** into a pot
- Bring to a boil
- Stir and <u>strain the water</u>
- Enjoy this drink while hot
- Repeat 3 times a day as needed

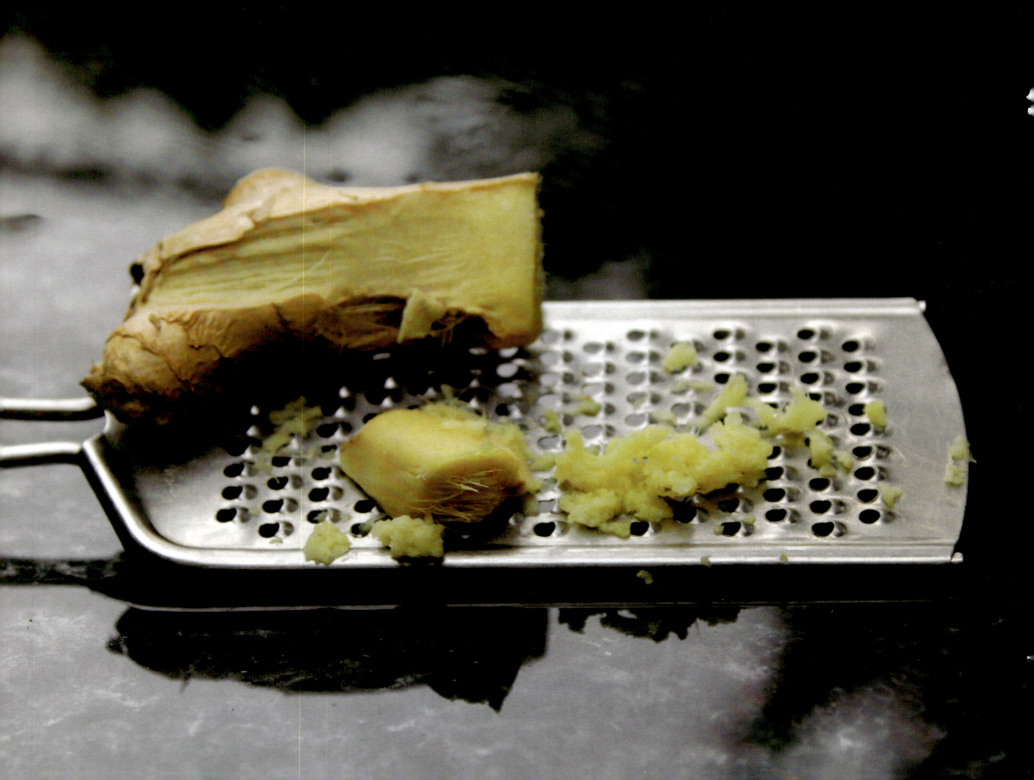

13. Āadunō Rus (Ginger Detox Juice)

આદુનો રસ

HELPS REMOVE TOXINS FOR COUGH, COLD, SINUS OR SORE THROAT

- Wash your hands

- Peel 1 inch fresh **GINGER**

- Grate the ginger

- Squeeze juice from the grated ginger into a bowl

- Add ¼ teaspoon of **SALT**

- Stir ingredients until salt has mixed in well and take ½ tablespoon

- Repeat daily as needed for relief

- <u>Avoid drinking water</u> for 30 minutes afterward

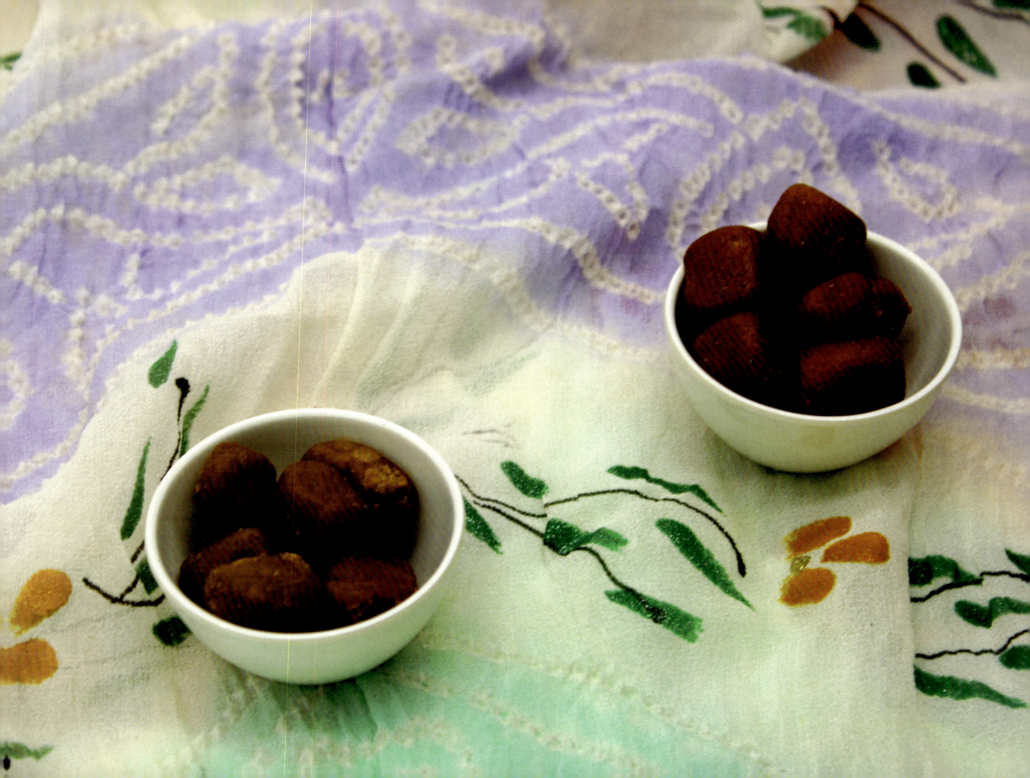

14. Soonṭh Pīprāmulnī Gōḷī (Ginger Donut Balls)

સૂંઠ પીપરામુલની ગોળી

TO CONTROL COUGH, COLD AND GAS

- In a small pan, heat 6 tablespoons of **PURE ORGANIC GHEE** on low flame

- Add 4 tablespoons (or ½ cup) grated **ORGANIC JAGGERY** and stir until jaggery melts

- <u>When jaggery melts, turn off stove</u> and quickly remove pan from the heat

- Transfer the melted jaggery to a plate

- Mix in 3 tablespoons of **PEEPRAMUL POWDER** and 1 tablespoon **GINGER POWDER**

- Stir ingredients well and let it cool

- Roll and shape into bite size donut balls of equal size

- Eat one daily after breakfast during winter season. Store the remaining ginger peepramul donut balls in an airtight container until ready to eat

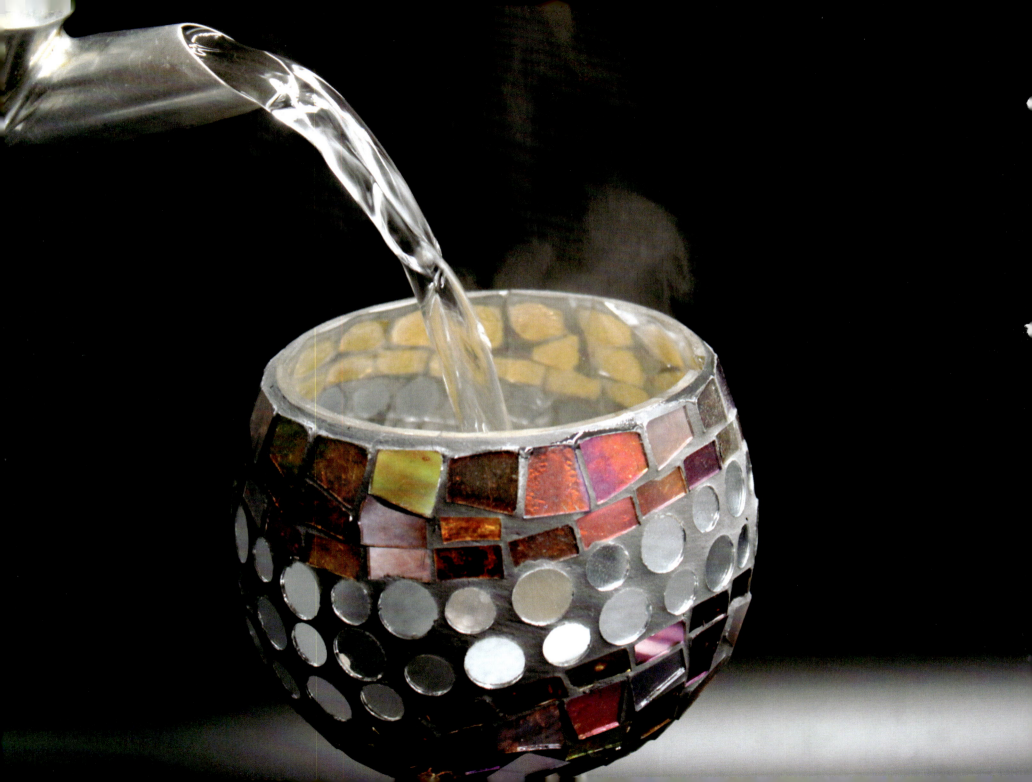

15. Garam Pāṇī Pīvānu (Hot Water Sips)

ગરમ પાણી પીવાનું

EXCELLENT FOR COLDS, ANTI-SEPTIC

- Add a cup of **WATER** to a pot on medium heat and let it heat for 2 minutes

- Turn off the heat and pour the hot water into a mug

- <u>Drink the water slowly while hot</u>

- Take deep breath for few seconds, then take sips again

- Repeat throughout the day to stay hydrated

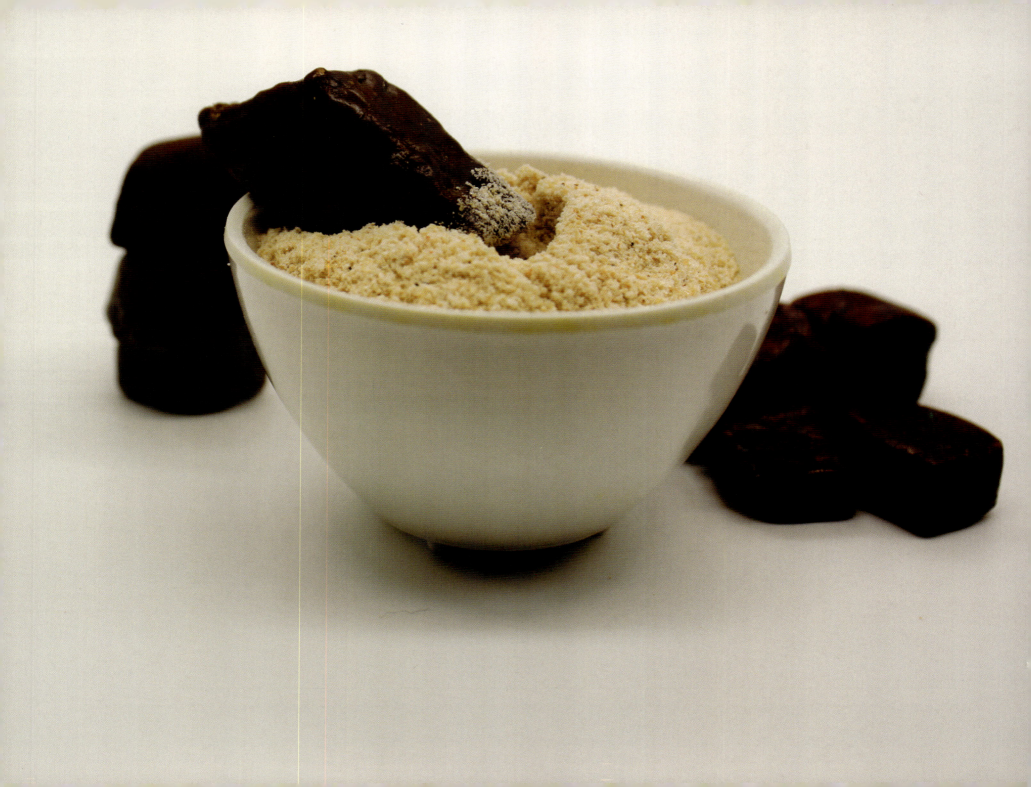

16. Hiṅg Chōpaḍvānu (Asafoetida Tummy Paste)

હિંગ ચોપડવાનું

TO PROVIDE RELIEF FOR TUMMY ACHE IN BABIES AND BABY COLIC

- Mix ¼ teaspoon of **ASAFOETIDA** with ¼-½ teaspoon of **WATER** to make a paste

- Using your fingertips, apply this paste on baby's tummy in a clockwise direction (about ¼-½ inch away from the bellybutton)

- Go in round circular motions around navel area (bellybutton) 3X

- The paste should <u>not touch the navel area</u>

- Let the paste dry

- Burp the baby to give relief from the gas and reduce tummy ache

- Wipe off the paste with a wet washcloth

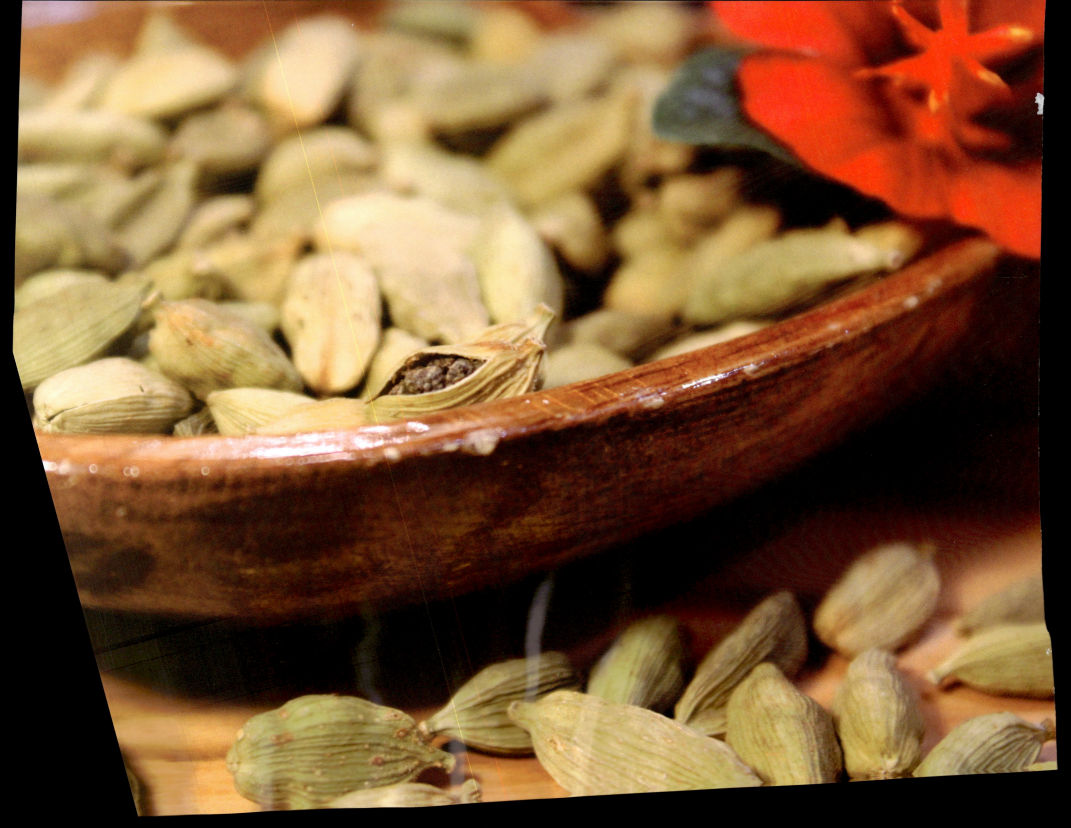

17. Elāichī anē Madh (Cardamom Honey Nectar)

ઇલાયચી અને મધ

To alleviate congestion and soothe from coughing

- Grind one <u>unshelled</u> **CARDAMOM POD** and one tiny **ROCK SALT** until they are pulverized into a fine powder

- Mix this in ¼ - ½ teaspoon of **ORGANIC HONEY**

- Add ½ - 1 teaspoon of **PURE ORGANIC GHEE** and mix well

- Eat this in the morning and at night as needed for relief

- <u>Avoid drinking water</u> for 30 minutes afterward

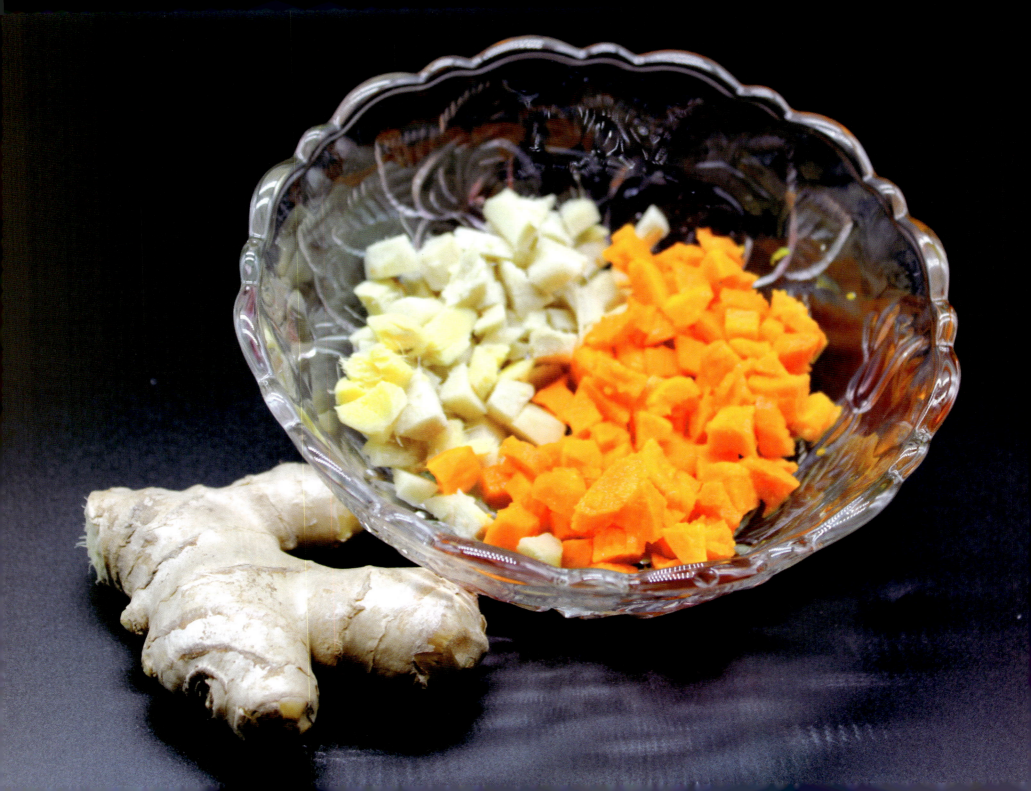

18. Ambā Haldarnō Ṭukaḍō (Mango Turmeric Gum)
આંબા હળદરનો ટુકડો

Helps suppress cough and fights chest congestion

- Peel ½ inch of **MANGO TURMERIC ROOT** and ½ inch of **TURMERIC ROOT**

- Dice in small pieces

- Add drops of **LEMON** and pinch of **SALT** (adjust per your taste)

- Chew one teaspoonful for few minutes until you absorb the juice then swallow

- Repeat this daily as needed

- Avoid drinking water for 30 minutes afterward

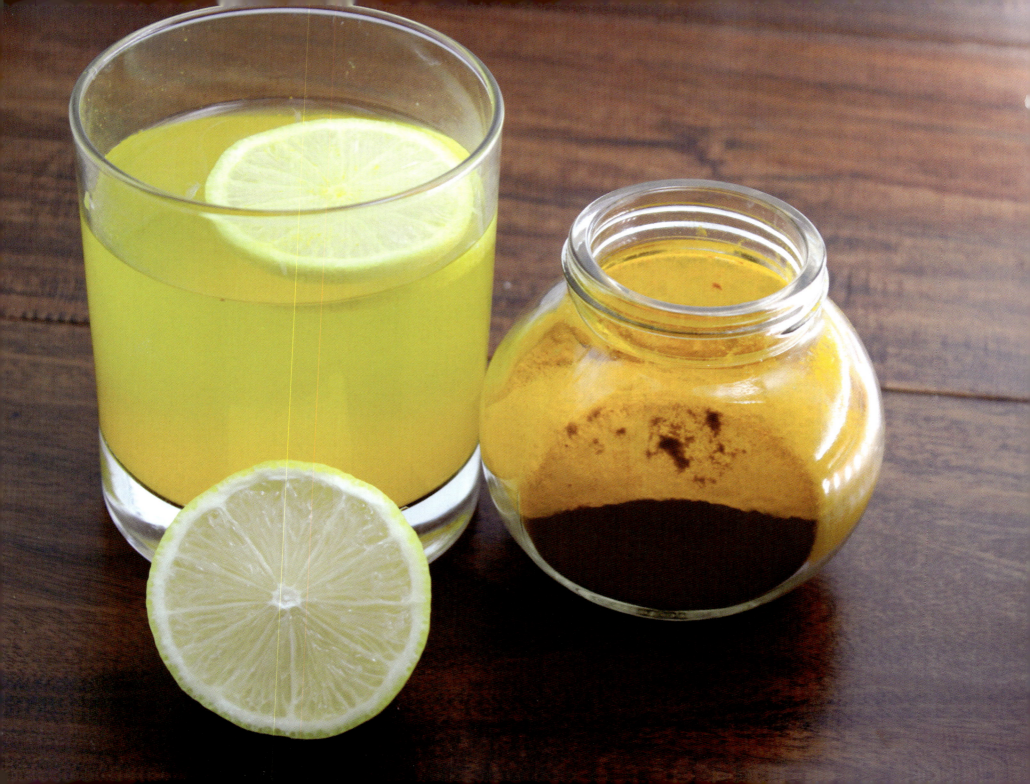

19. Haḷdar Līmbunu Pāṇī (Turmeric Detox)

હળદર લીંબુનું પાણી

USEFUL FOR CONSTIPATION

- Heat an 8 ounces glass of **WATER** in a small pot on medium flame

- Add ¼ teaspoon **GROUND ORGANIC TURMERIC POWDER**

- Cut 1 fresh **LEMON** into four quarters

- Squeeze juice from 1 quarter lemon or ½ teaspoon size

- Sprinkle a pinch of **SALT** to taste

- Mix thoroughly and remove from the heat after 2 minutes

- Enjoy this warm beverage by drinking it slowly first thing in the morning on an empty stomach <u>before brushing teeth</u>

- Repeat daily as needed

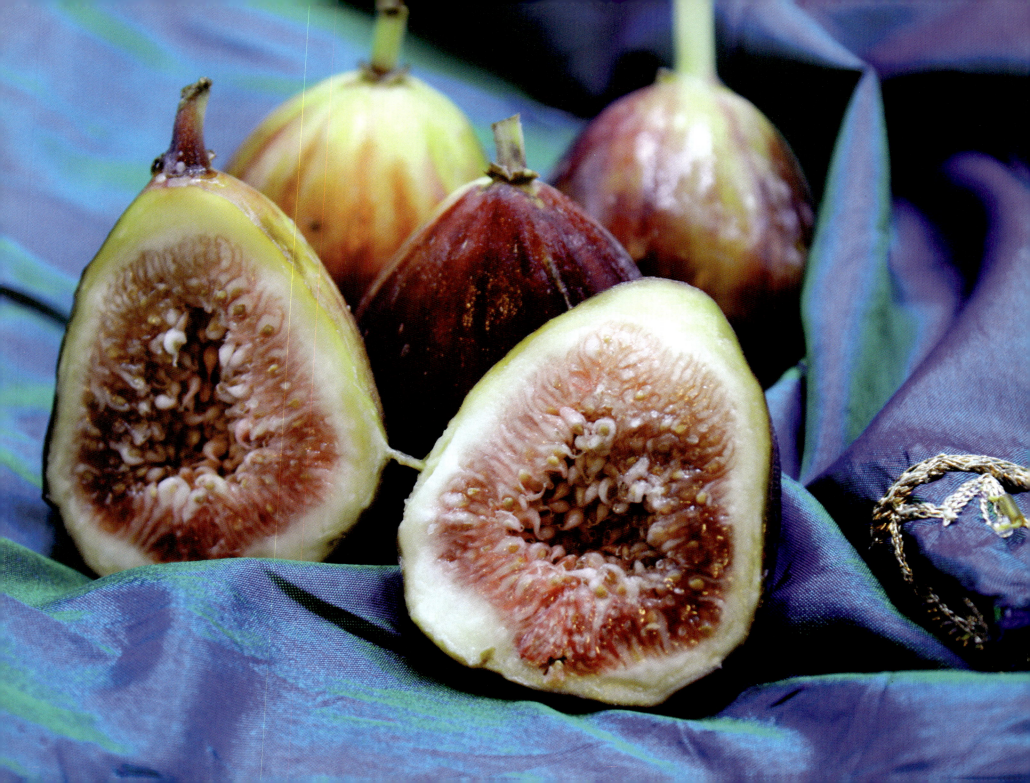

20. Anjeer (Fiber Rich 'n Regular Figs)

અંજીર

HELPS TO RELIEVE CONSTIPATION

- Soak 2 **DRIED FIGS** <u>overnight</u> in 4 ounces glass of **WATER** and cover with a lid

- Optional to add: soak 10 **BLACK RAISINS** overnight to same glass of water as dried figs

- In the morning strain the water to a small bowl and eat the figs on an empty stomach

- Drink the strained water

- Repeat daily as needed

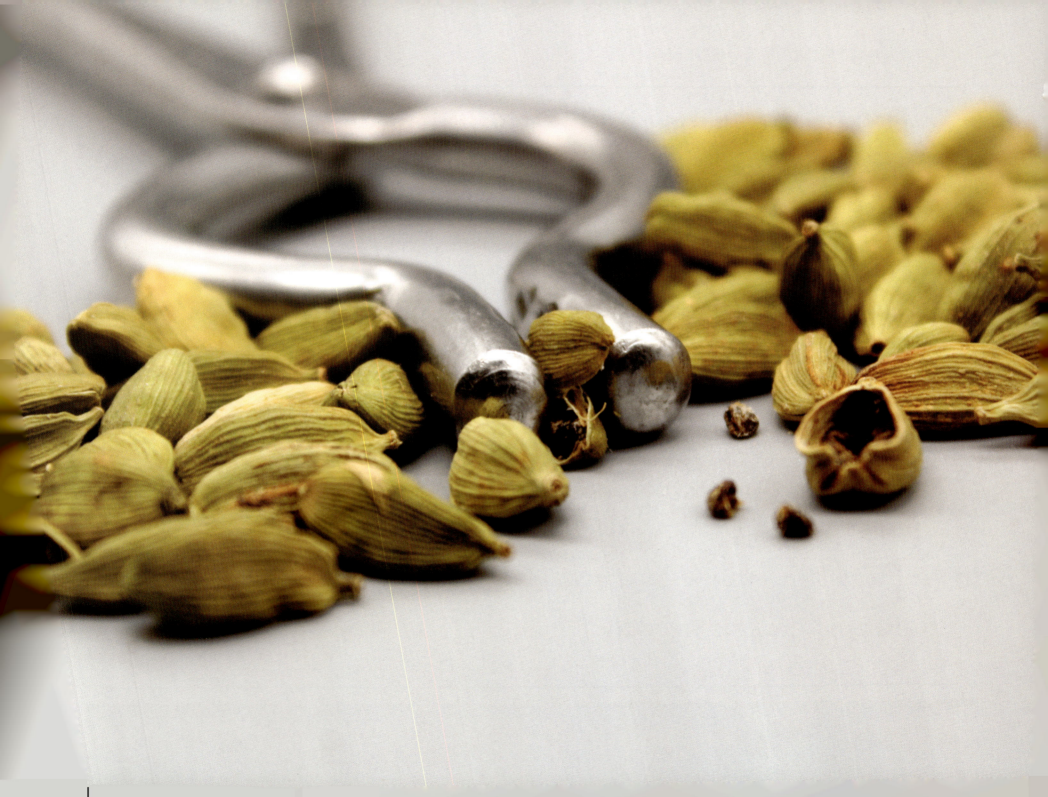

21. Elāichīnā Fōtrā (Roasted Cardamom Pod Syrup)
ઇલાયચીના ફોતરા

HELPS TO FIGHT DRY COUGH

- Roast outer shell of **CARDAMOM POD** by holding it under a flame for 6-8 seconds. Use a tong to hold the pod when roasting
- Let it cool and open the shell
- Grind cardamom seeds using a rolling board and rolling pin until pulverized into a fine powder
- Heat ½ teaspoon of **PURE ORGANIC GHEE** over low flame until it melts
- In a small bowl, add the melted ghee and mix with powdered cardamom and 1 teaspoon of **ORGANIC HONEY**
- Pour into a spoon and enjoy this fine flavorful syrup
- Consume this 3 times a day as needed
- Avoid drinking water for 30 minutes afterward

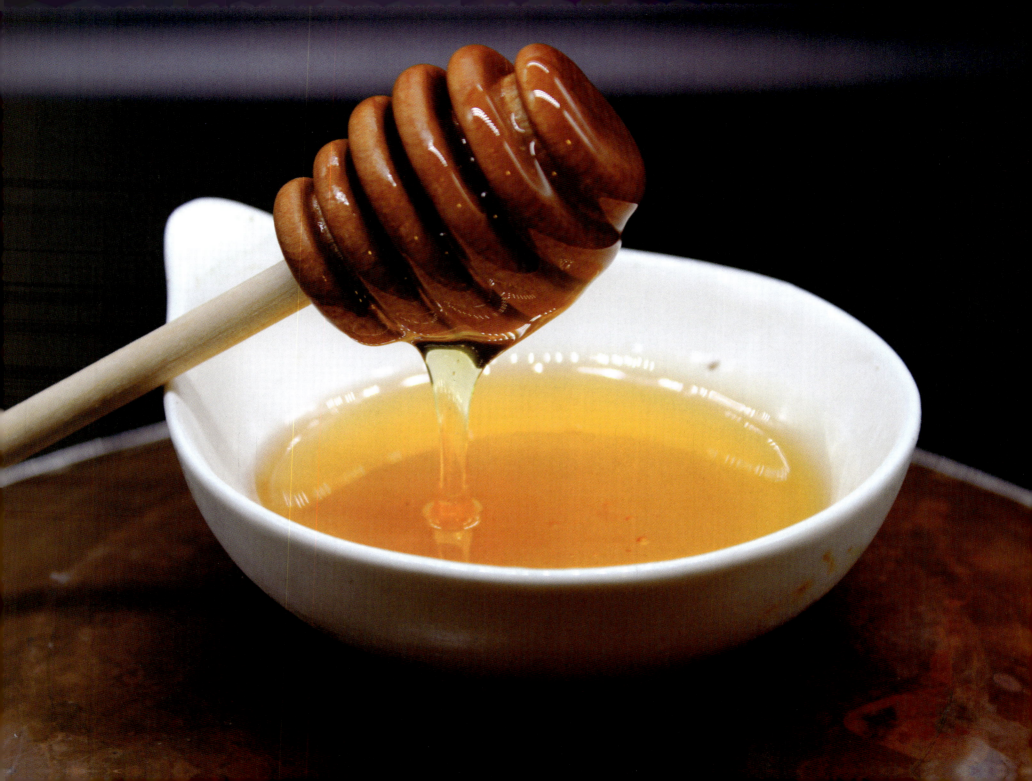

22. Madh anē Līmbu (Honey Lemon Drop)

મધ અને લીંબુ

TO ALLEVIATE DRY COUGH

- Cut 1 fresh **LEMON** into four quarters

- Squeeze two drops of fresh lemon juice from 1 quarter lemon into 1 tablespoon of **ORGANIC HONEY**

- Drink this after each meal or 3 times a day

- <u>Avoid drinking water</u> for 30 minutes after taking this solution

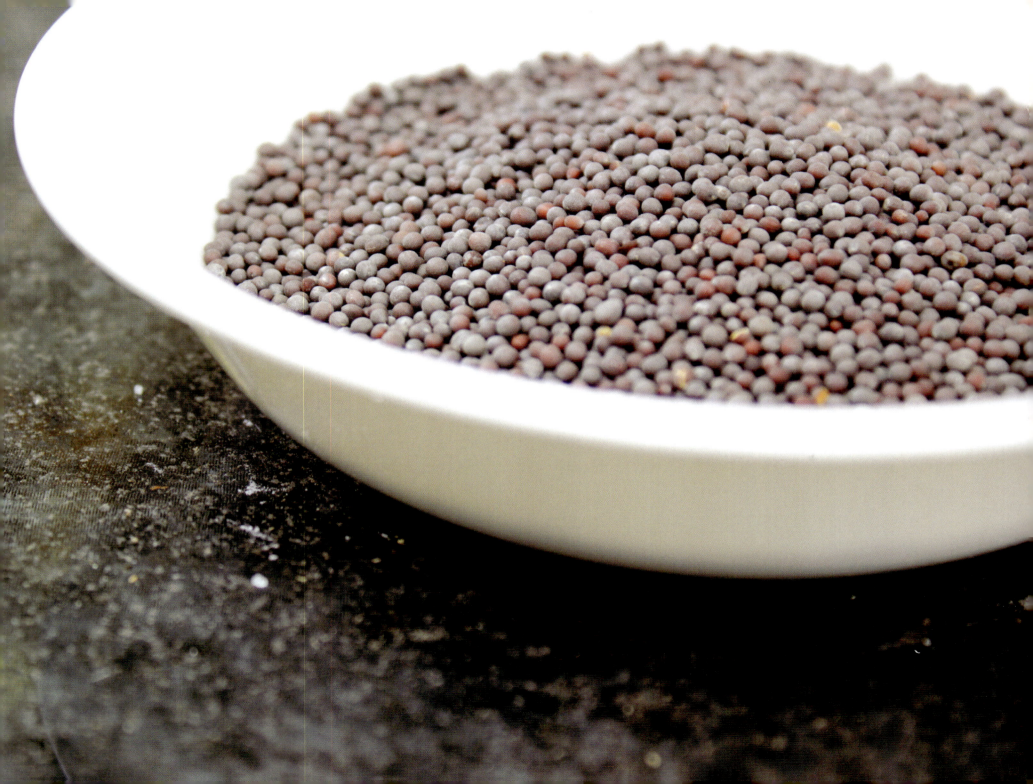

23. Rā'īnu Pāṇī (Mustard Seeds Drink)
રાઈનું પાણી

TO ALLEVIATE COUGH SYMPTOMS

- Grind 1 teaspoon of **MUSTARD SEEDS** into a fine powder

- Mix this powder in 8 ounces **LUKEWARM WATER**

- Let steep for 15 minutes

- Pour ¼ cup dose in a glass and enjoy this drink

- Repeat throughout the day as needed

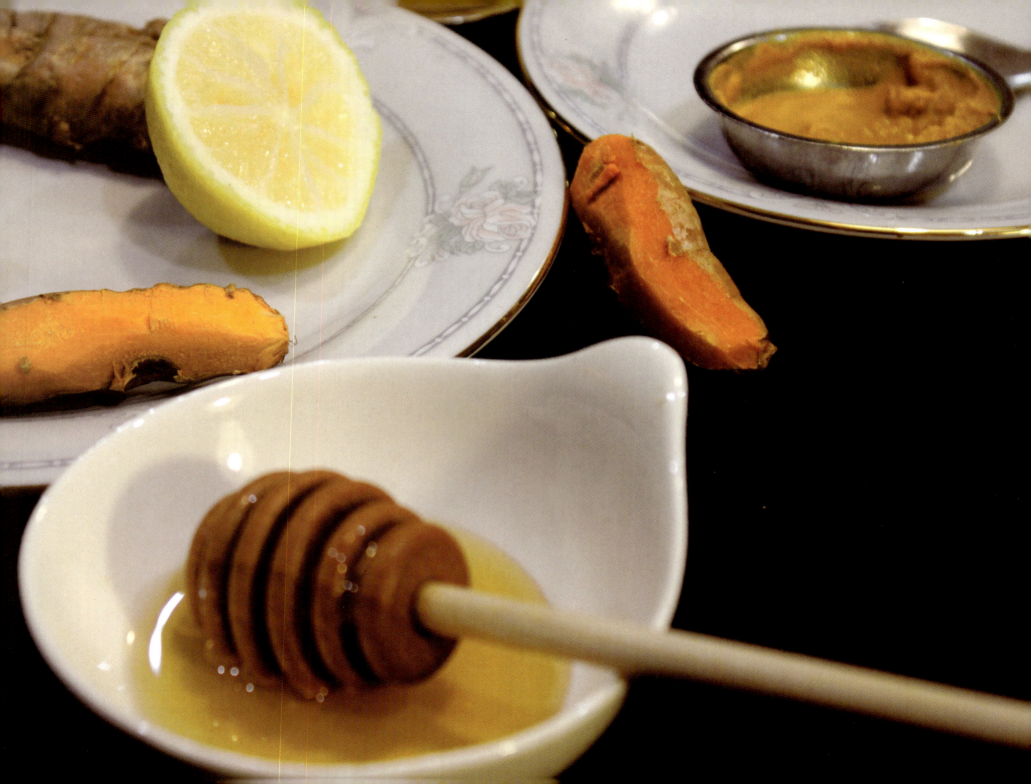

24. Madh anē Haḷdar (Turmeric Honey Elixir)
મધ અને હળદર

TO SUPPRESS COUGHING

- Warm 1 teaspoon of **ORGANIC HONEY** over the stove (for small children, reduce to ½ teaspoon of honey)

- Add a pinch of **GROUND ORGANIC TURMERIC POWDER**

- Combine and stir this mixture

- Consume one teaspoonful

- Avoid drinking water for 30 minutes after taking this solution

- Take this three times a day (after each meal) as needed

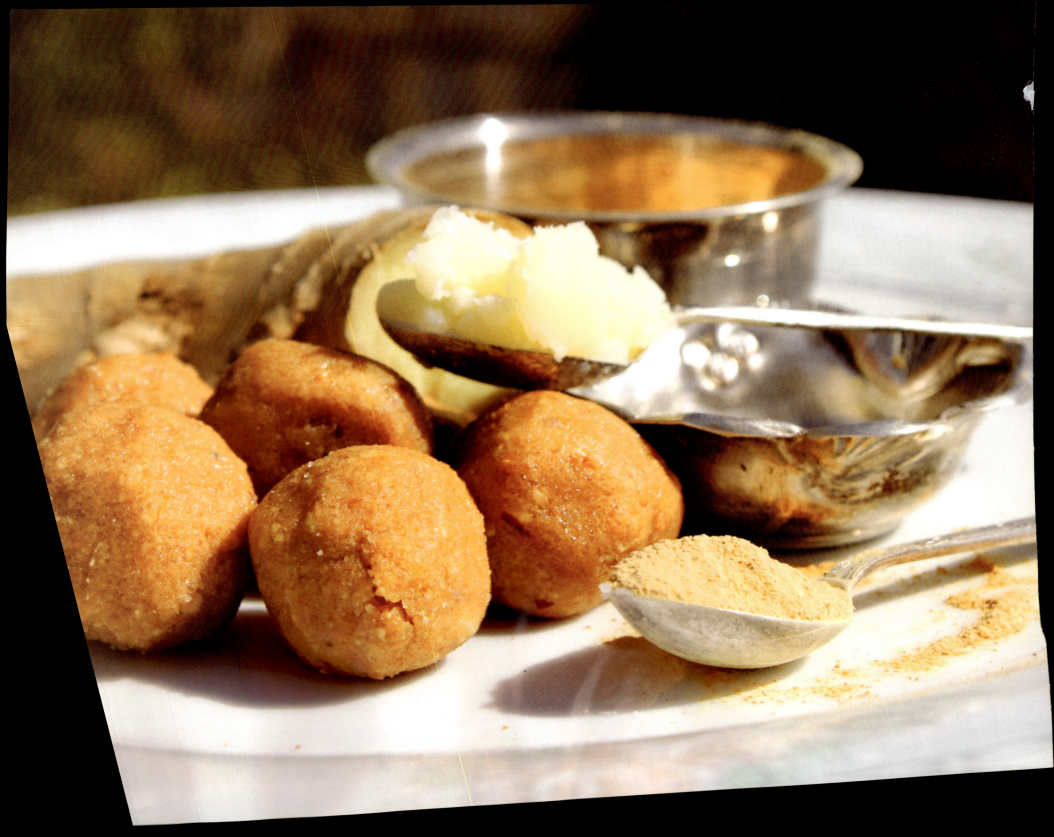

25. Soonthnī Lāḍuḍī (Immune Boosting Balls)

સૂંઠની લાડુડી

To alleviate cough symptoms

- Heat 2 tablespoons of **PURE ORGANIC GHEE** in a small pan over low flame
- When ghee melts, add 1½ teaspoon sliced **ORGANIC JAGGERY**
- <u>When jaggery melts, turn off stove</u> and quickly remove pan from the heat
- Transfer the melted jaggery to a plate
- Mix in 1 teaspoon of **GINGER POWDER**
- After it cools, make into smooth doughy paste
- Roll into bite size mini-balls of equal size
- Store in an airtight container
- Eat one daily as needed

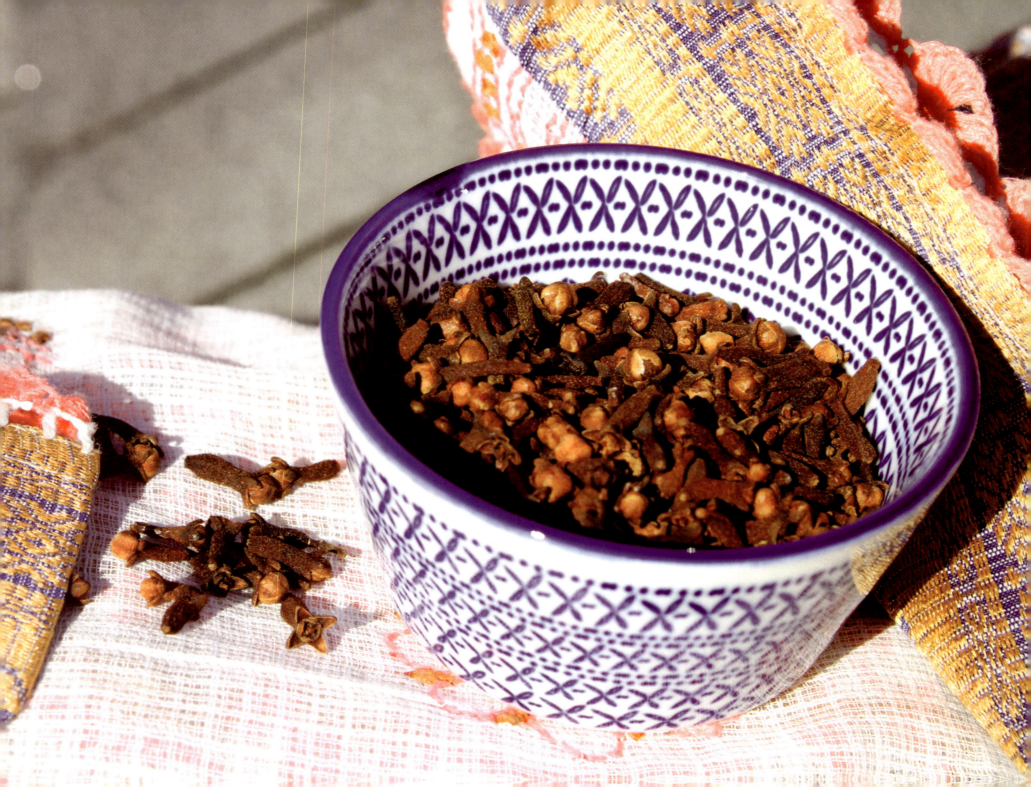

26. Śhēkēlu Lavīṅg (Roasted Clove Drops)
શેકેલું લવીંગ

HELPS TO FIGHT COUGH

- Remove the bud (top section) from one **CLOVE**

- Roast the clove stem by holding it under a flame for 8-10 seconds. Use a tong to hold the clove when roasting

- Let it cool

- Suck on it without chewing to get as much of the flavor

- Then chew and swallow it

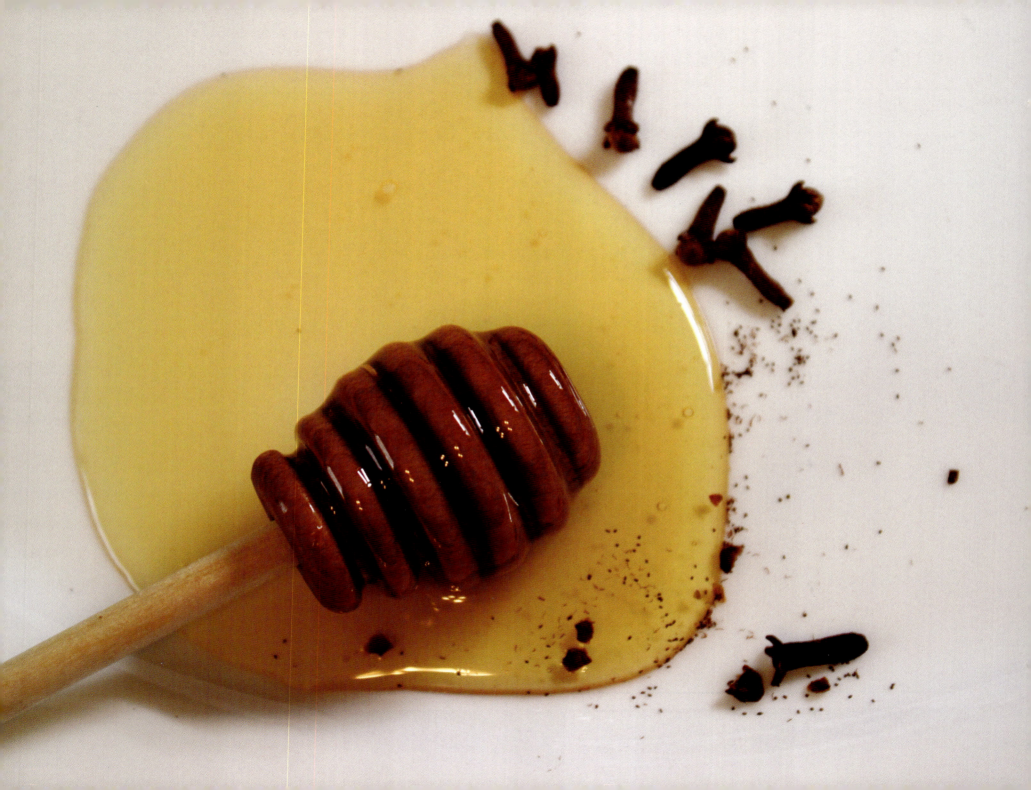

27. Lavīṅg anē Madh (Clove Infused Honey)

લવીંગ અને મધ

Helps to fight cough

- Remove the bud (top section) of 5 **CLOVES**

- Grind the clove stems until pulverized into a fine powder

- Mix this with a teaspoon of **ORGANIC HONEY**

- Put this in mouth and slowly swallow

- Enjoy this flavored warming concoction in the morning and at night

- <u>Avoid drinking water</u> for 30 minutes after eating this

- Repeat 2 times a day as needed

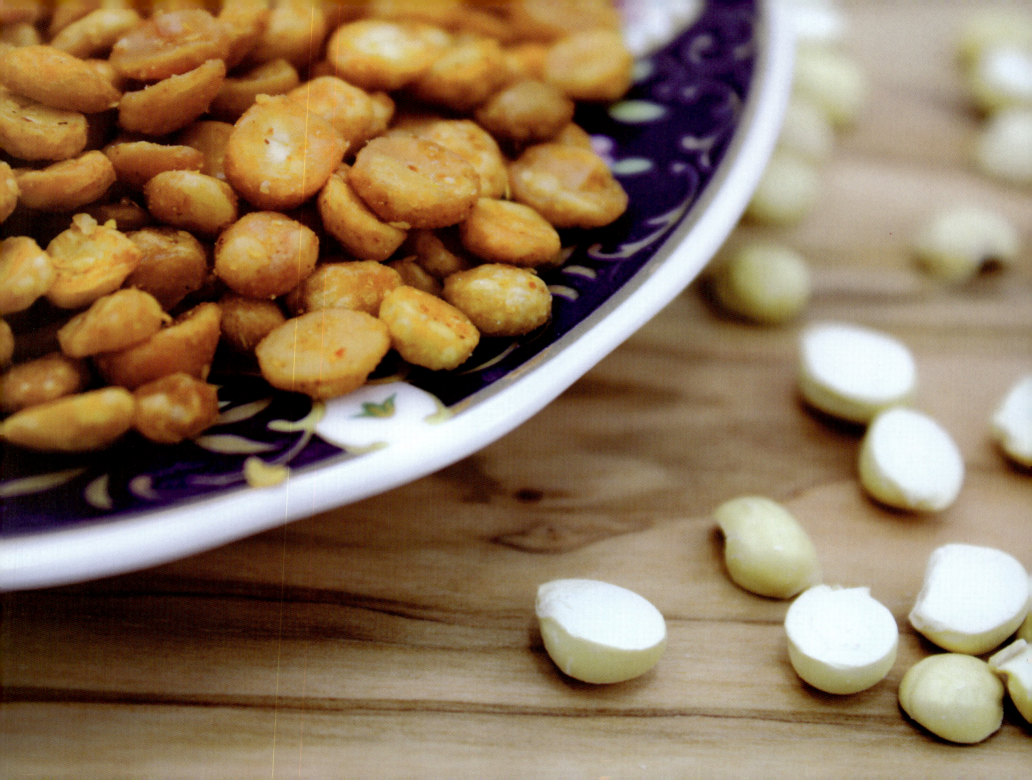

28. Dāḷiā (High-Protein Roasted Chana)
દાળીયા

USEFUL FOR COUGH

- Eat **PLAIN ROASTED CHANA** without skin (or roasted chana with **TURMERIC POWDER** and **SALT**) before going to bed

- Avoid drinking water for 30 minutes after eating

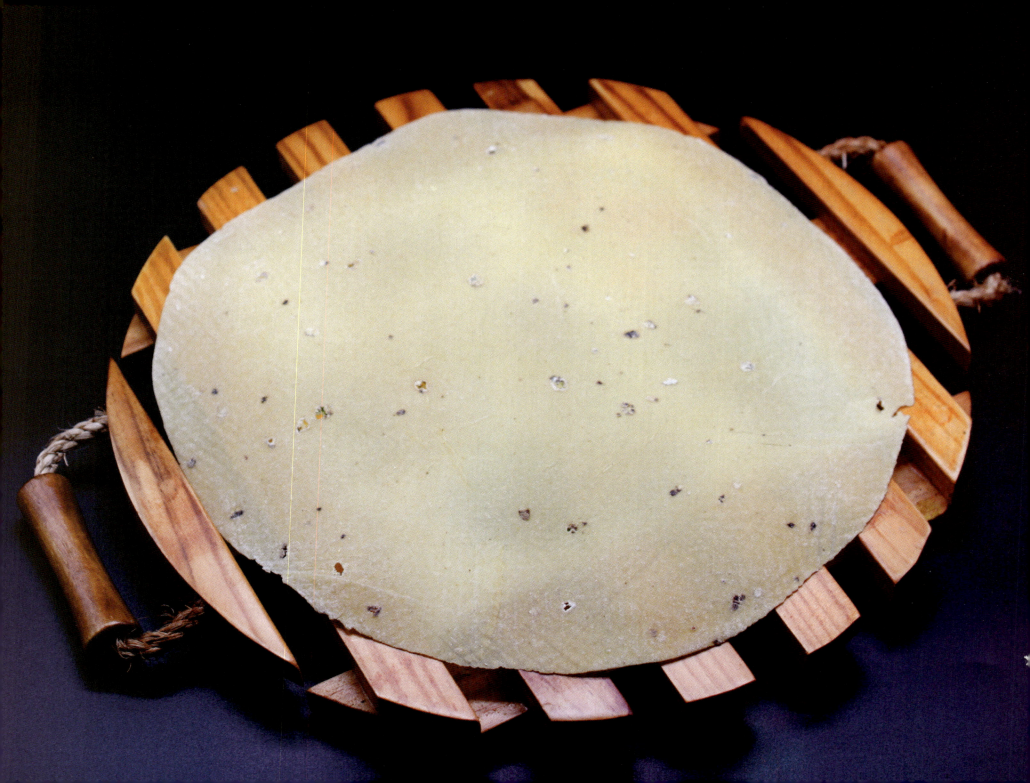

29. Kāchō Pāpaḍ (Unroasted Raw Papadum)
કાચો પાપડ

TO ALLEVIATE NIGHTTIME COUGH SYMPTOMS

- Cut 1 raw (<u>dried but not roasted</u>) **PLAIN PAPADUM** into 8 equal pieces

- Chew on 1-2 pieces slowly before going to bed (store the remaining pieces in an airtight container)

- Do not drink water after that

- Repeat nightly as needed

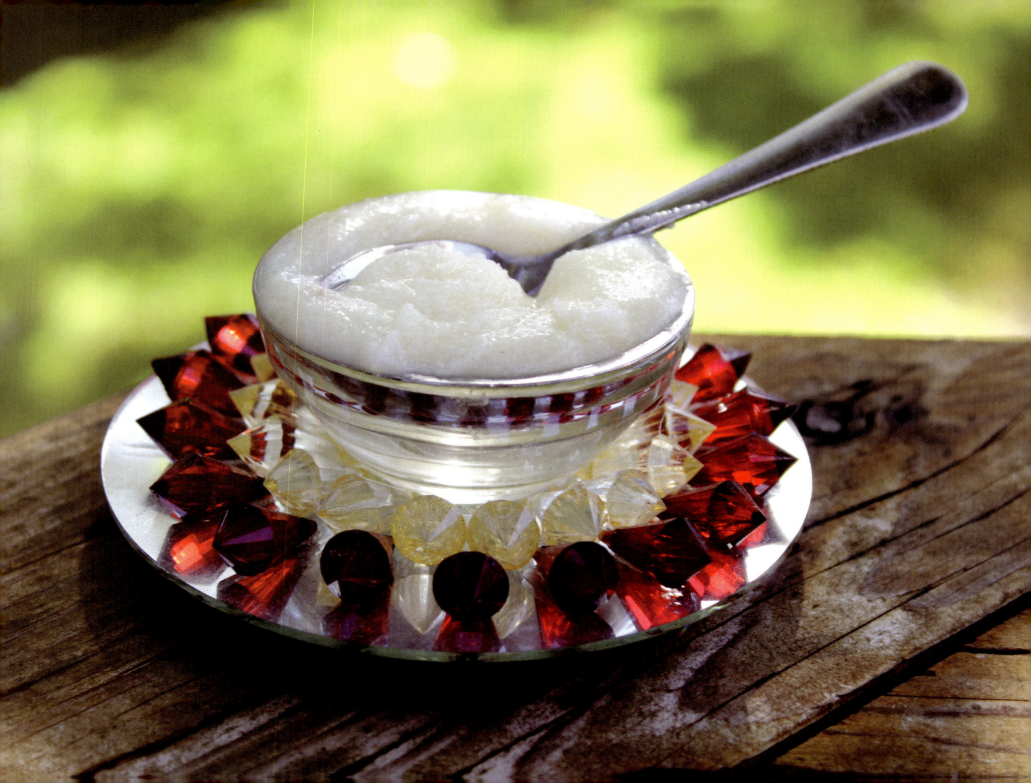

30. Āṅkhō Māṭe Gheenu Māliśh (Ghee Eye Massage)

આંખો માટે ઘીનું માલિશ

REDUCE DARK CIRCLES UNDER EYES

- Before going to bed, take 1 drop of **PURE ORGANIC GHEE** on your fingertip

- Rub the fingers to warm the ghee

- Gently rub ghee on the dark circle skin area under your eyes

- Avoid getting in your eyes

- Massage the area gently for 1 minute

- Let it stay overnight

- Rinse with **WATER** in the morning

- Repeat daily

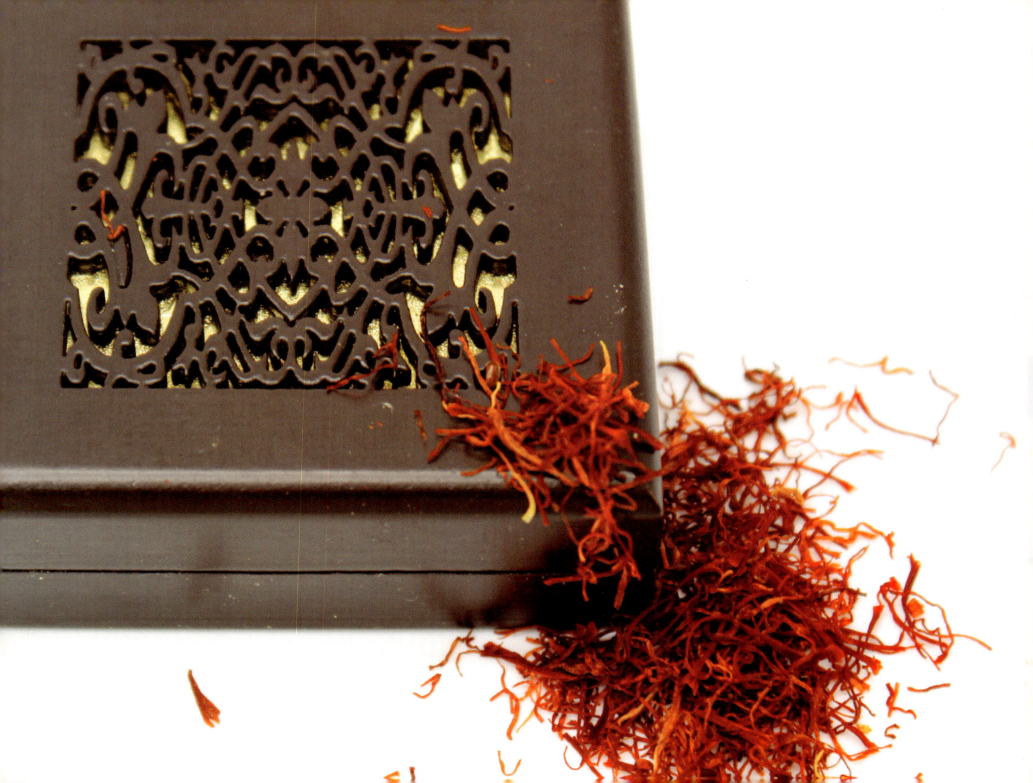

31. Kēsarnu Māliśh (Saffron Eye Mask)

કેસરનું માલિશ

REDUCE DARK CIRCLES UNDER EYES

- Wash your hands
- Take 4 small threads of **ORGANIC SAFFRON** and gently crush to a powder state using your fingers
- Soak powdered saffron in ¼ cup **MILK** of your choice for 5 minutes
- Dip a cotton ball to soak the saffron-infused milk
- Apply this eye mask on the dark circle area under eye area (note: avoid getting saffron paste inside the eye as it can cause irritation)
- Leave it for 10 minutes
- Rinse with water
- Repeat once a week

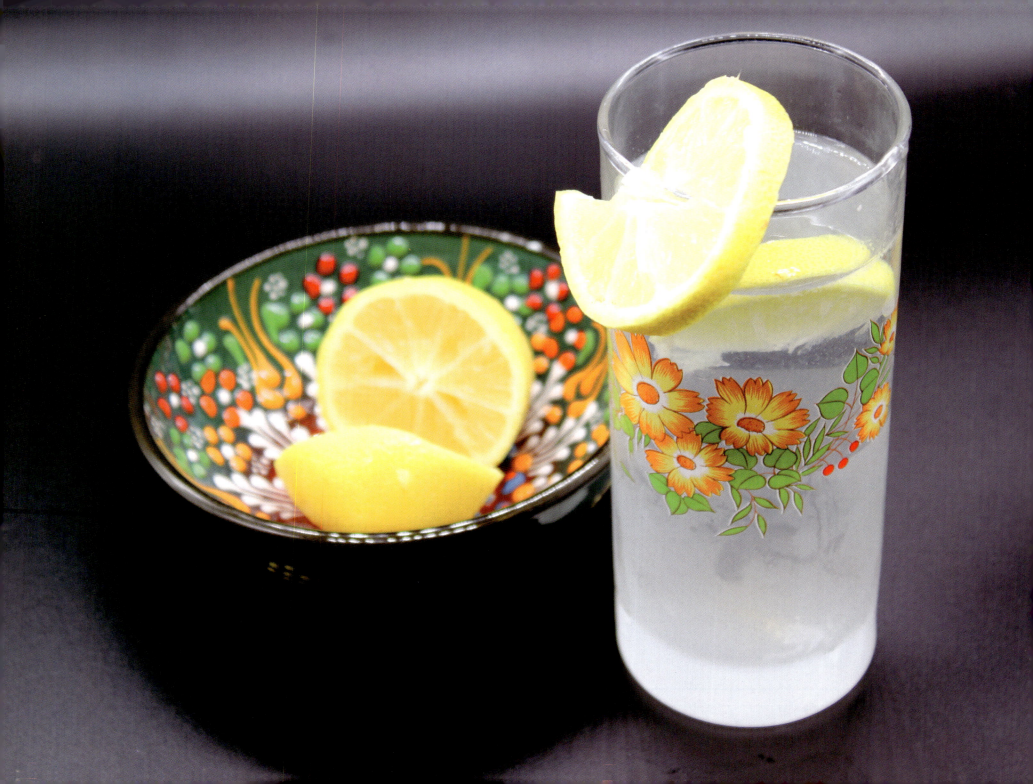

32. Līmbunu Śharbat (Thirst Quencher Lemonade)

લીંબુનું શરબત

IMPROVE DEHYDRATION AND BOOSTS ELECTROLYTES

- Pour **WATER** in an 8 ounce glass

- Squeeze 1 medium **LEMON** (2 tablespoons of juice)

- Add 2-3 tablespoons of your preferred **SUGAR**

- Add a pinch of **SALT** and pinch of **GROUND BLACK PEPPER POWDER**

- Mix all the ingredients well

- Enjoy this cooling, refreshing drink

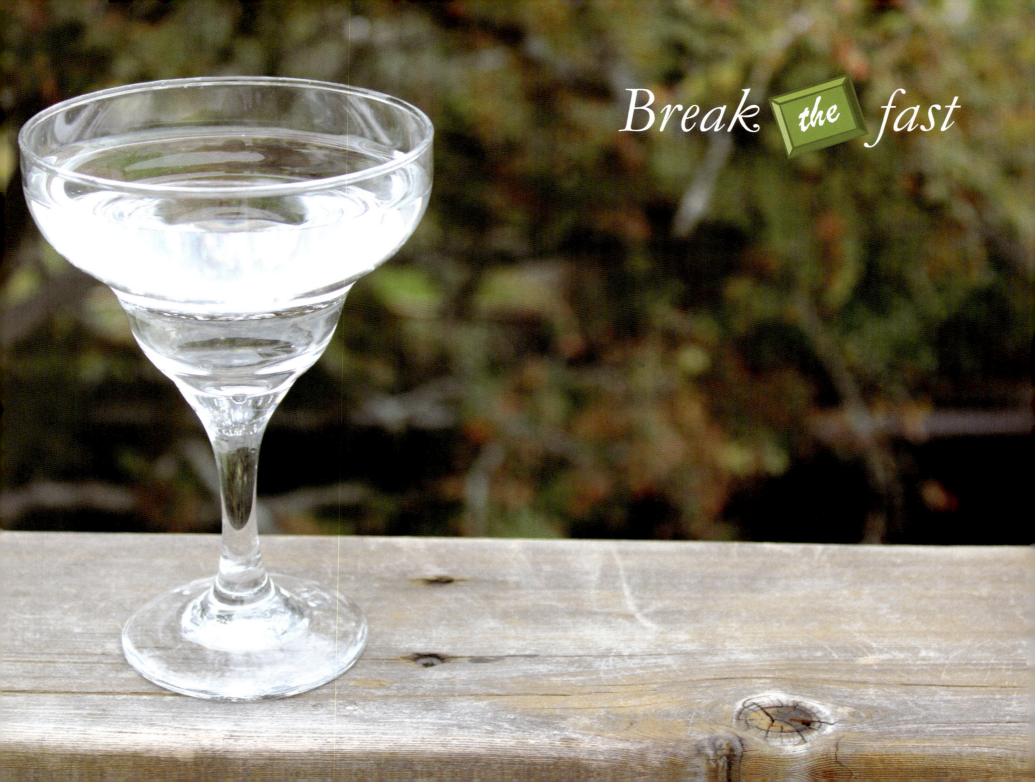

Break *the* fast

33. Upvās (Self-Discipline 1-Day Water Fast)
ઉપવાસ

DETOXIFICATION & IMMUNITY BOOST

1. **Day Before the 1-Day Fast**
- Stop eating at least 48 minutes before sunset
2. **During the 1-Day Fast**
- Drink boiled water only - no food, juice, coffee/tea
- Boil a pot of **WATER** in the morning
  - Strain water and let it cool in a covered jug
  - Do not leave in refrigerator
  - Drink water – 64 oz/day
    - From 48 minutes past sunrise
    - Until 48 minutes before sunset
  - Fast the entire day
  - Rest as needed
  - By sunset throw out any unused water

3. **Day After the Fast**
- Boil a pot of water in the morning
- Break the fast gently 48 minutes after sunrise (known as "Parna")
- Start with sipping light, simple drinks
  - Khaḍī Sāakar (Remedy 41)
  - Gōḷnu Pāṇī (Remedy 70)
  - Lavīṅgnu Pāṇī (Remedy 71)
  - Gundarnī Rāab (Remedy 72)
  - Moongnu Pāṇī (Remedy 88)
  - Saākarnu Pāṇī (Remedy 92)
- Introduce milder foods such as Moong (Remedy 88)
- Add solid foods & increase fiber to your diet slowly
- After you break the fast, be extra cautious and eat less than you normally would for that day

Fasting may not be suitable for everyone.
Do what is comfortable for you.

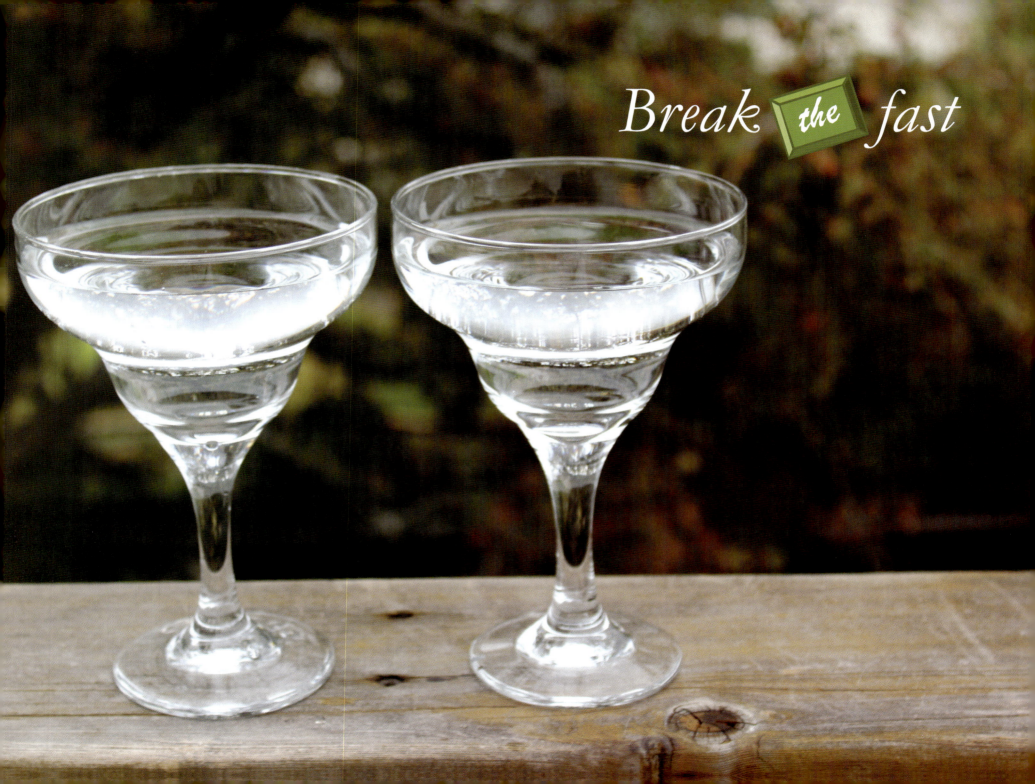

Break *the* fast

34. Chhaṭh (Power Pack 2-Days Water Fast)

૬૪

DETOXIFICATION & IMMUNITY BOOST

1. **Day Before the 2-Day Fast**
- Stop eating at least 48 minutes before sunset

2. **During the 2-Day Fast**
- Drink boiled water only - no food, juice, coffee/tea
- Boil a pot of **WATER** in the
  - Strain water and let it cool in a covered jug
  - Do not leave in refrigerator
  - Drink water– 64 oz/day
    - From 48 minutes past sunrise
    - Until 48 minutes before sunset
- Fast the entire day
- Rest as needed
- By sunset throw out any unused water

3. **Day After the Fast**
- Boil a pot of water in the morning
- Break the fast gently 48 minutes after sunrise (known as "Parna")
- Start with sipping light, simple drinks
  - Khaḍī Sāakar (Remedy 41)
  - Gōḷnu Pāṇī (Remedy 70)
  - Lavĭṅgnu Pāṇī (Remedy 71)
  - Gundarnī Rāab (Remedy 72)
  - Moongnu Pāṇī (Remedy 88)
  - Sāakarnu Pāṇī (Remedy 92)
- Introduce milder foods such as Moong (Remedy 88)
- Add solid foods & increase fiber to your diet slowly
- After you break the 2-day fast, be extra cautious and eat less than you normally would for next 2 days

Fasting may not be suitable for everyone.
Do what is comfortable for you.

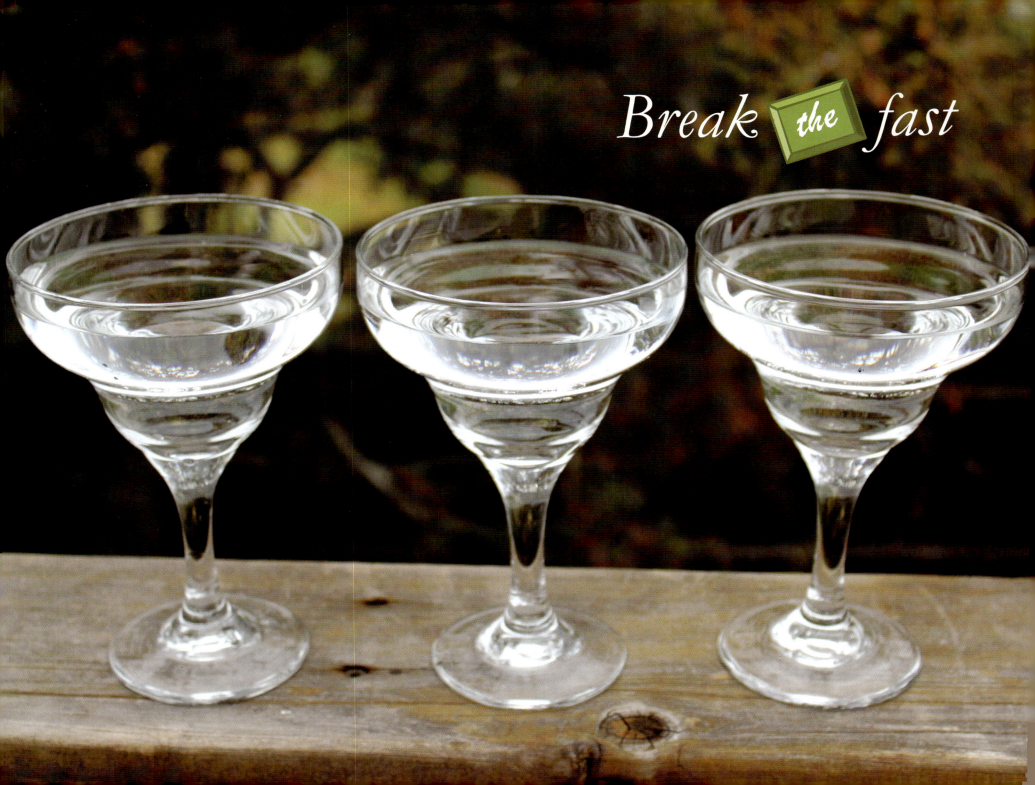

Break *the* fast

35. Aṭtham (Transformational 3-Days Water Fast)
અઠ્ઠમ

AUTOPHAGY, DETOXIFICATION & IMMUNITY BOOST

1. **Day Before the 3-Day Fast**
- Stop eating at least 48 minutes before sunset

2. **During the 3-Day Fast**
- Drink boiled water only - no food, juice, coffee/tea
- Boil a pot of **WATER** in the morning
  - Strain water and let it cool in a covered jug
  - Do not leave in refrigerator
  - Drink water – 64 oz/day
    - From 48 minutes past sunrise
    - Until 48 minutes before sunset
  - Fast the entire day
  - Rest as needed
  - By sunset throw out any unused water

3. **Day After the Fast**
- Boil a pot of water in the morning
- Break the fast gently 48 minutes after sunrise (known as "Parna")
- Start with sipping light, simple drinks
  - Khaḍī Sāakar (Remedy 41)
  - Gōḷnu Pāṇī (Remedy 70)
  - Laviṅgnu Pāṇī (Remedy 71)
  - Gundarnī Rāab (Remedy 72)
  - Moongnu Pāṇī (Remedy 88)
  - Sāakarnu Pāṇī (Remedy 92)
- Introduce milder foods such as Moong (Remedy 88)
- Add solid foods & increase fiber to your diet slowly
- After you break the 3-day fast, be extra cautious and eat less than you normally would for next 3 days

> *Fasting may not be suitable for everyone.*
> *Do what is comfortable for you.*

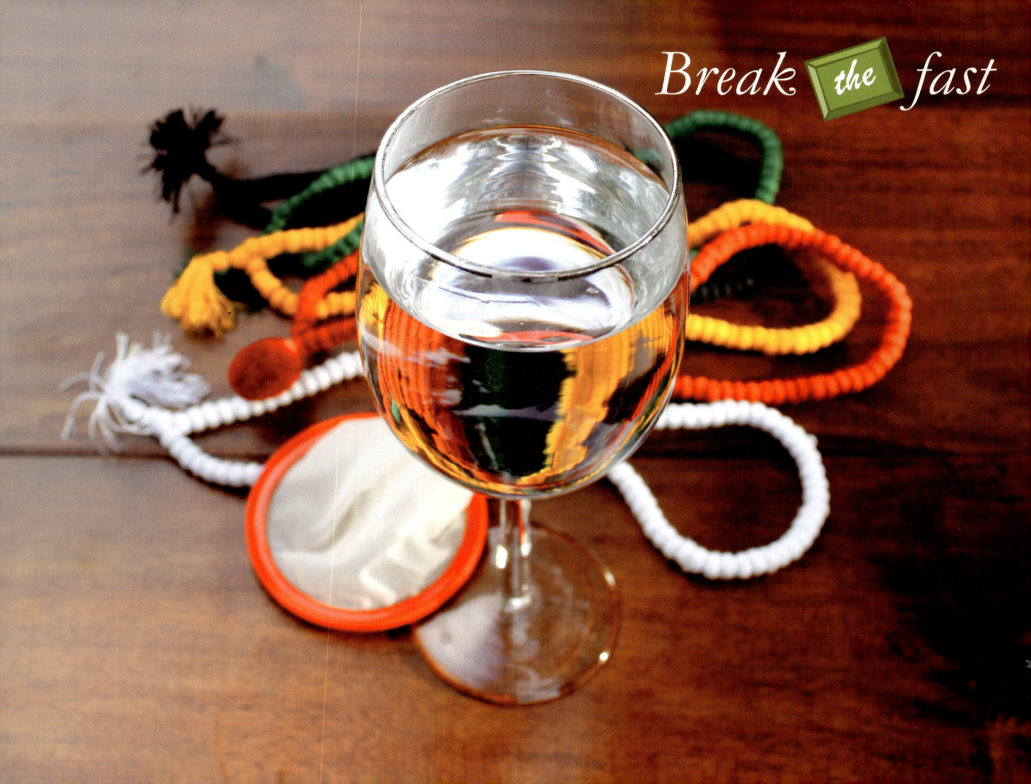

Break *the* fast

36. Āyambīl (Forever Cleanse for Victory over Taste)
આયંબીલ

DETOXIFICATION, CONQUER PHYSICAL APPETITE & THE MIND, BALANCE DIGESTIVE SYSTEM

1. **Day Before Āyambīl**
   - Stop eating at least 48 minutes before sunset

2. **During Āyambīl**
   - Drink boiled water (follow steps on how to boil water as shown in Remedy 33)

3. **One Time Sitting Meal during day of Āyambīl**
   - Eat food once per day in one sitting anytime from 48 minutes after sunrise and complete by 48 minutes before sunset.

4. **The Day After Āyambīl**
   - Follow steps in Remedy 33 as shown in the section "Day After the Fast"

5. **Food Restrictions during the day of Āyambīl**
   - List of foods to refrain from
     - Vegetables (including Green, Raw, Root)
     - Dairy Products including Milk, Butter, Ghee
     - Processed/Stale/Frozen
     - Fermented
     - Sugar/Jaggery
     - Oil/Fried
     - Fruits
     - Honey, Spices*
   - Example of plain foods to consume
     - Freshly Prepared Chapati (Indian Roti)
     - Boiled/Cooked Rice, Grains
     - Moong Beans, Lentils
     - Khichadi
     - Following spices* are allowable during Āyambīl:
       - Āyambīl Asafoetida
       - Āyambīl Salt
       - Āyambīl Black Pepper

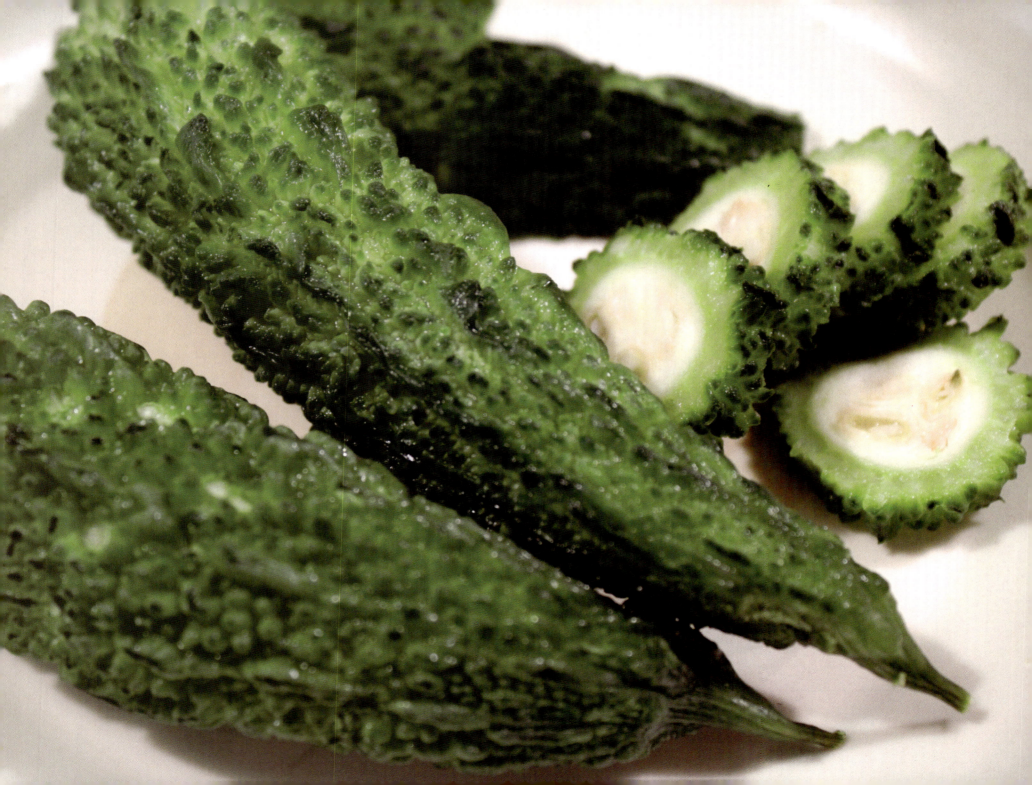

37. Kārēlānō Rus (Reverse Diabetes Smoothie)

કારેલાનો રસ

To control and manage diabetes, regulate blood sugar level

- Thoroughly wash 1 small, fresh **BITTER GOURD**
- Remove both ends of the bitter gourd
- Cut the vegetable in the center. Remove any large seeds
- Chop into small pieces and put to a bowl. Add ½ teaspoon of **SALT** of your choice and ½ cup of **WATER** to the bowl.
- Let it soak for 30 minutes, then place chopped bitter gourd and the water into a blender
- Cut 1 medium **LEMON** into quarters, and squeeze one quarter of juice into bowl
- Add ¼ teaspoon of **GROUND ORGANIC TURMERIC POWDER** and blend the ingredients until juice is smooth
- Strain the pulp from the blender into a medium size bowl using a metal sieve and a spoon. Slowly add ½ cup of water to help extract the juice
- Add a pinch of **GROUND BLACK PEPPER POWDER** and salt to taste
- Stir well and pour the juice immediately into a serving glass
- Enjoy this beverage <u>first thing in the morning</u> on an empty stomach

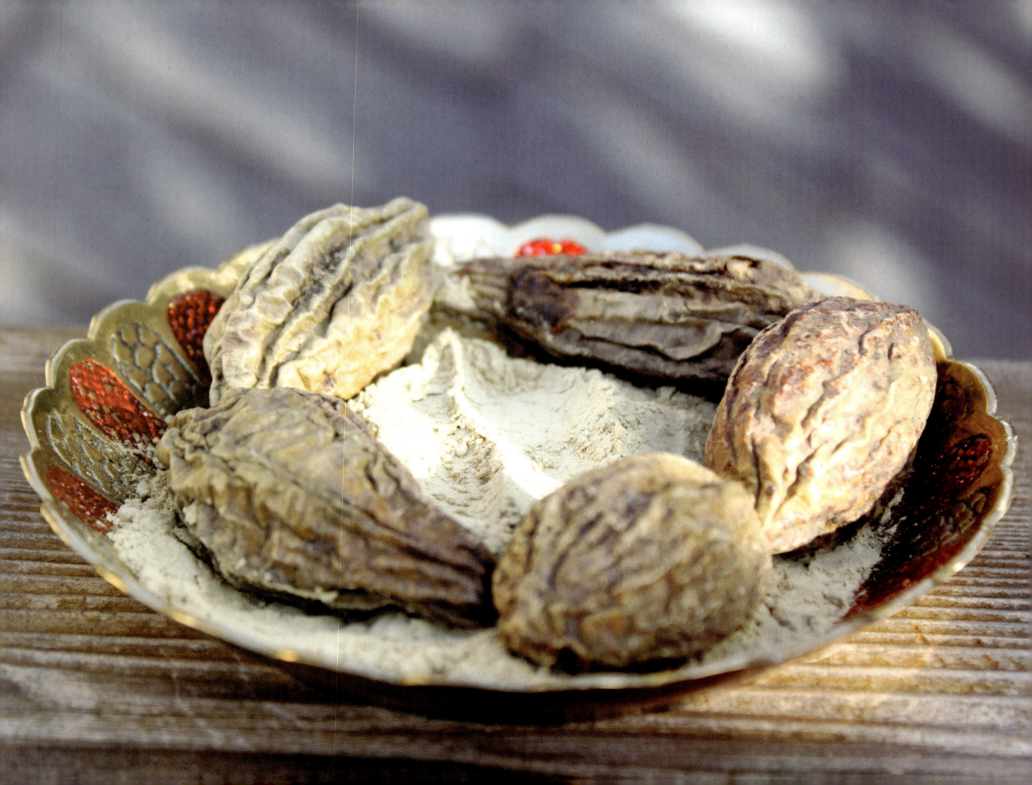

38. Harḍēnu Pāṇī (Diabetes Dried Superfruit)

હરડેનું પાણી

FOR DIABETES PREVENTION, CONTROLS BLOOD SUGAR LEVEL, HELPS IN WEIGHT LOSS

- Heat 1 cup of **WATER** in a small pot on medium flame
- Immediately before the water comes to a boil, turn off the heat
- Add ½ teaspoon of **HARDE POWDER** (also known as **HARITAKI POWDER**)
- Mix well (optional: add a drop of **ORGANIC HONEY** to the mixture)
- Pour into a mug, cover with a lid and let it cool
- Enjoy this beverage <u>2 hours after you finish dinner</u>

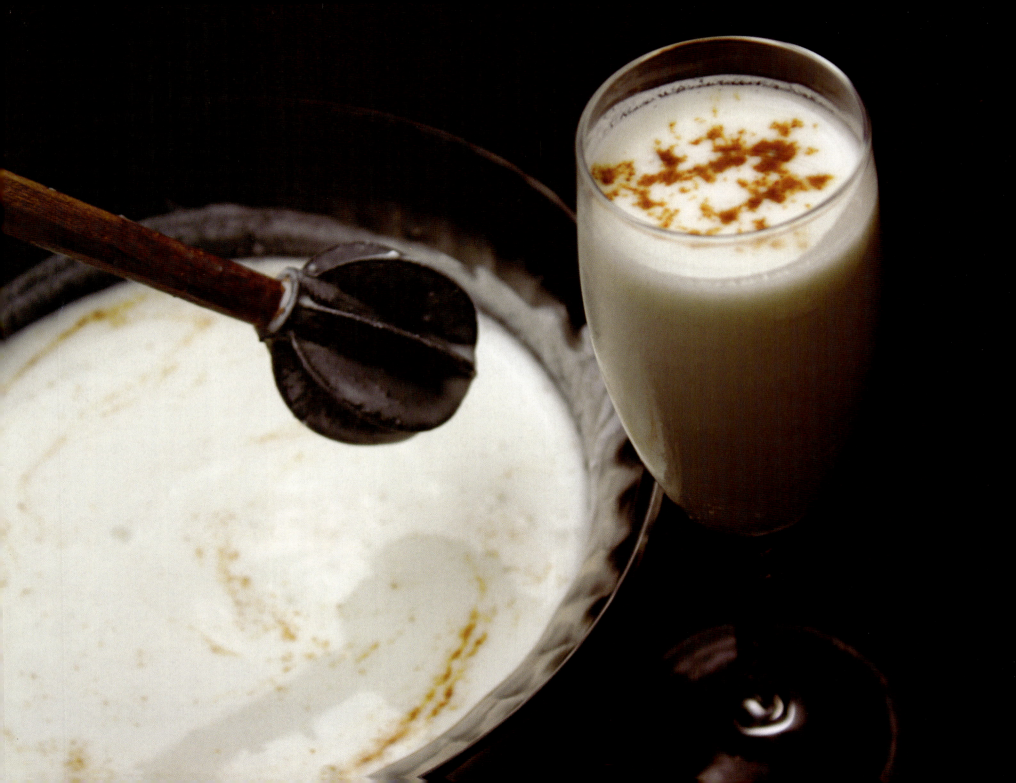

39. Las'sī (Relaxing Yogurt Beverage)

લસ્સી

To Alleviate diarrhea

- In a large bowl add ½ cup of plain **YOGURT** of your choice
- Add ½ cup of **WATER**
- Roast 1 teaspoon organic **CUMIN SEEDS** and grind to a fine powder
- Add roasted, powdered cumin seeds
- Add ¼ teaspoon of **SALT** (adjust quantity as per your taste)
- Whisk the ingredients well
- Pour in a glass and drink

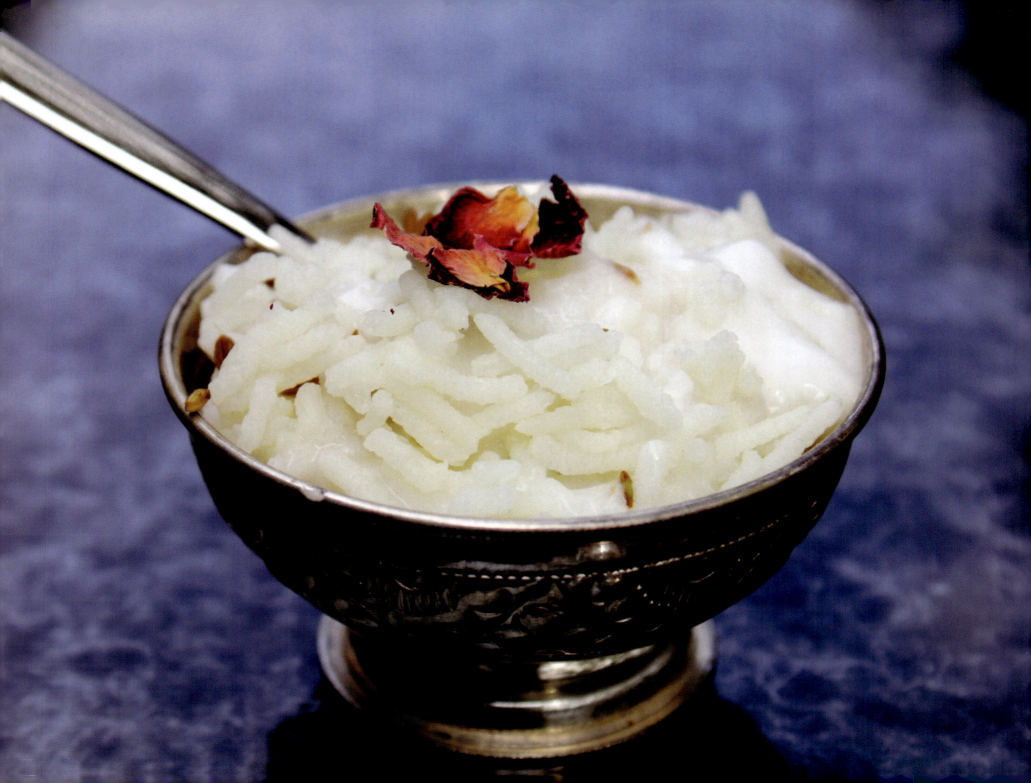

40. Dahī anē Bhāat (Comfort Curd Rice)

દહી અને ભાત

To Alleviate diarrhea

- Soak ¼ cup of your preferred long-grain **RICE** in water for 30 minutes and then drain the water

- Add ½ cup of **WATER** in small pot on medium heat

- When it comes to a boil, add rice with pinch of **SALT**

- Let the rice overcook to a mushy, sticky porridge consistency

- In a large bowl, add ¼ cup of plain **YOGURT** of your choice

- Add the cooked rice

- Add 1 tablespoon **PURE ORGANIC GHEE**

- Mix the ingredients until well combined

- Serve into a bowl and enjoy this comfort rice

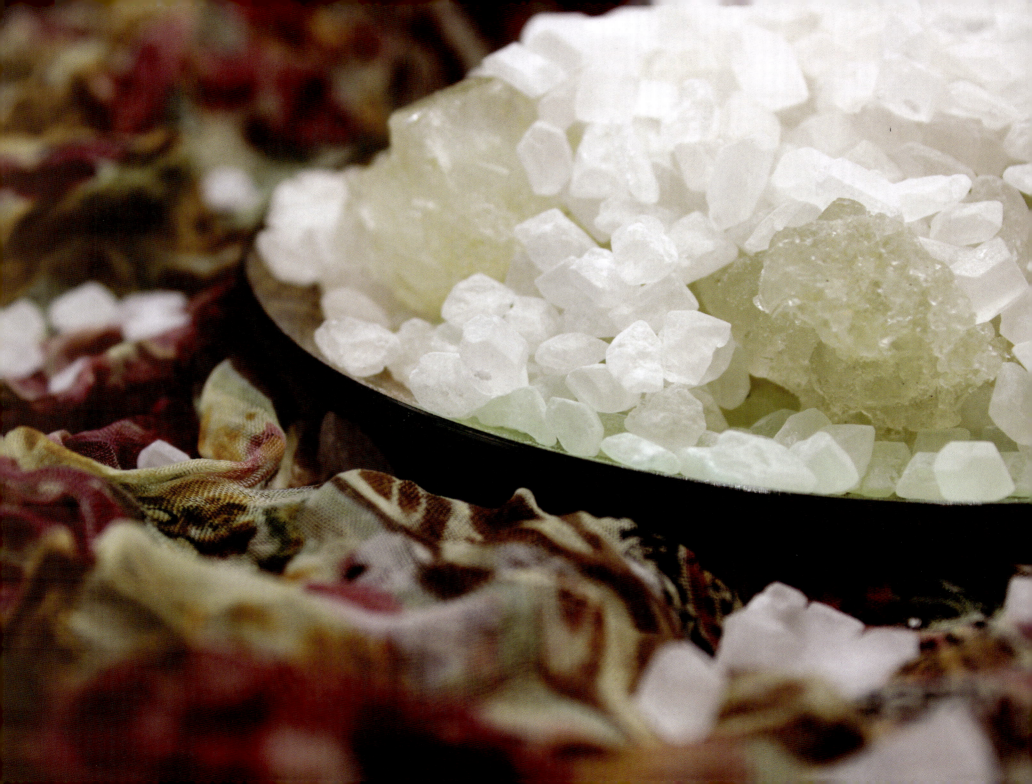

41. Khaḍī Sāakar (Rock Sugar Drink)
ખડી સાકર

To Alleviate diarrhea

- Add 1 cup of **WATER** to a small pot

- Bring to a boil

- Add 2 small **ROCK SUGARS** to boiling water

- Mix until <u>sugar melts</u> and then turn off heat

- Pour into a bowl and stir well

- Enjoy this drink while hot

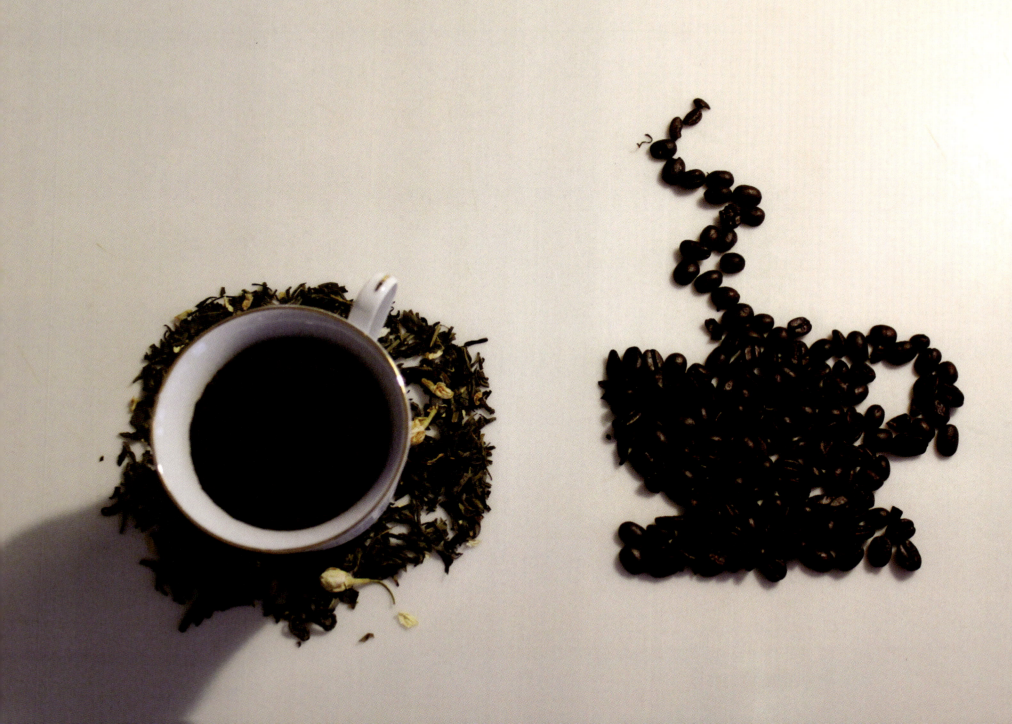

42. Kāḷī Chā | Kōphee (Black Tea or Coffee)
કાળી ચાય | કોફી

To Alleviate diarrhea

- Boil 1 cup **WATER**

- Add 1 teaspoon of **BLACK TEA** or **COFFEE**

- Let it boil to ½ of its original proportion

- Filter and pour in a mug

- Enjoy this drink while hot

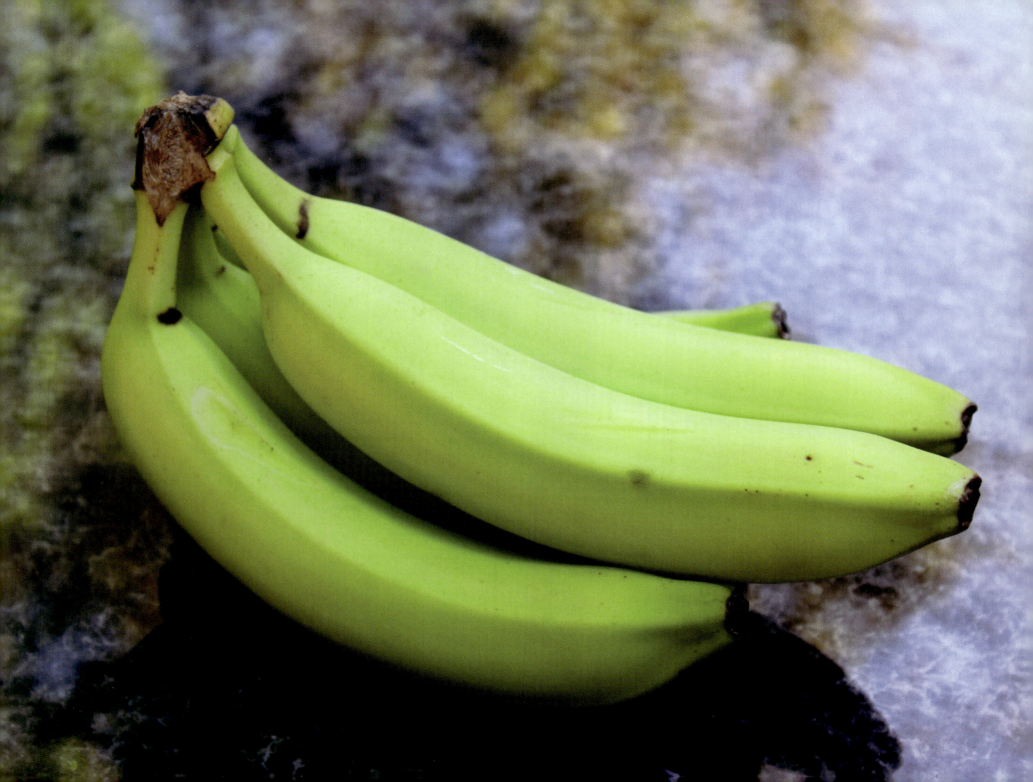

43. Kāchā Kēḷā (Unripe Green Banana)

કાચા કેળા

To Alleviate diarrhea

* Eat 1 <u>unripe</u> **GREEN BANANA**

* Repeat next day as needed

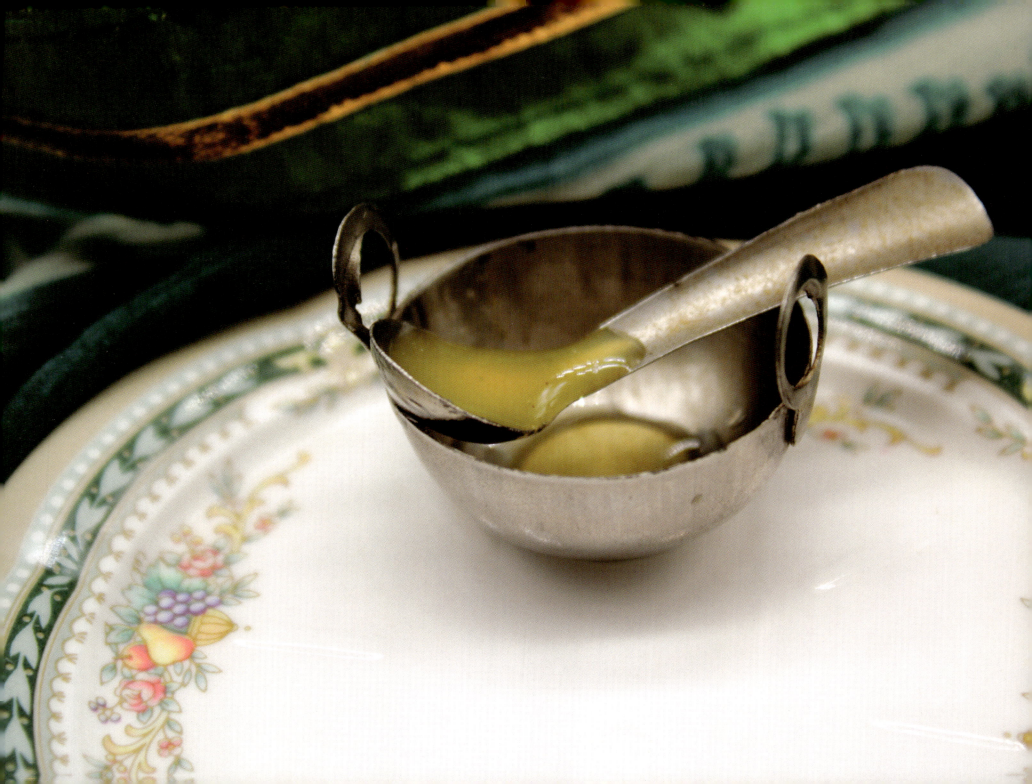

44. Gheenu Pāṇī (Gut Soother)

ઘીનું પાણી

IMMEDIATE RELIEF FROM CONSTIPATION, AIDS DIGESTION

- Heat 1 glass of **WATER** in a pot

- Add 1 teaspoon of **PURE ORGANIC GHEE**

- Add pinch of **SALT**

- Stir well

- Drink this water <u>slowly</u> first thing in the morning on an empty stomach

- If needed repeat before going to bed, at least one hour after dinner

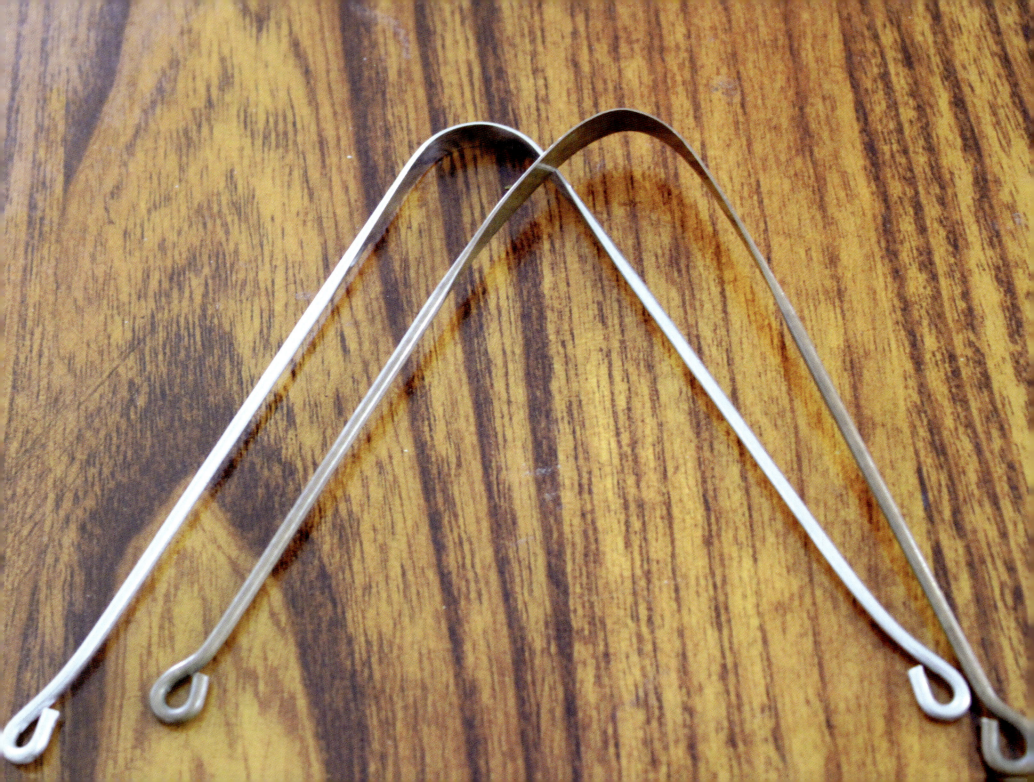

45. Ūlīyu (Tongue Scraper)

ઊલીયુ

AIDS IN DIGESTION AND ORAL HEALTH, REMOVES BACTERIA, REDUCES BAD BREATH

- Drink 2 glasses of **LUKEWARM WATER** on an empty stomach first thing in the morning, then do the following

- Brush your teeth, gargle and rinse

- While standing in front of a mirror, stick out your tongue

- Hold a **TONGUE SCRAPER** using both hands as far back on your tongue as possible

- Gently <u>scrape forward</u> and rinse off the white film coating on your tongue 1-2 times

- After scraping your tongue, rinse the tongue scraper with hot water and your mouth with water

- Repeat this morning routine daily

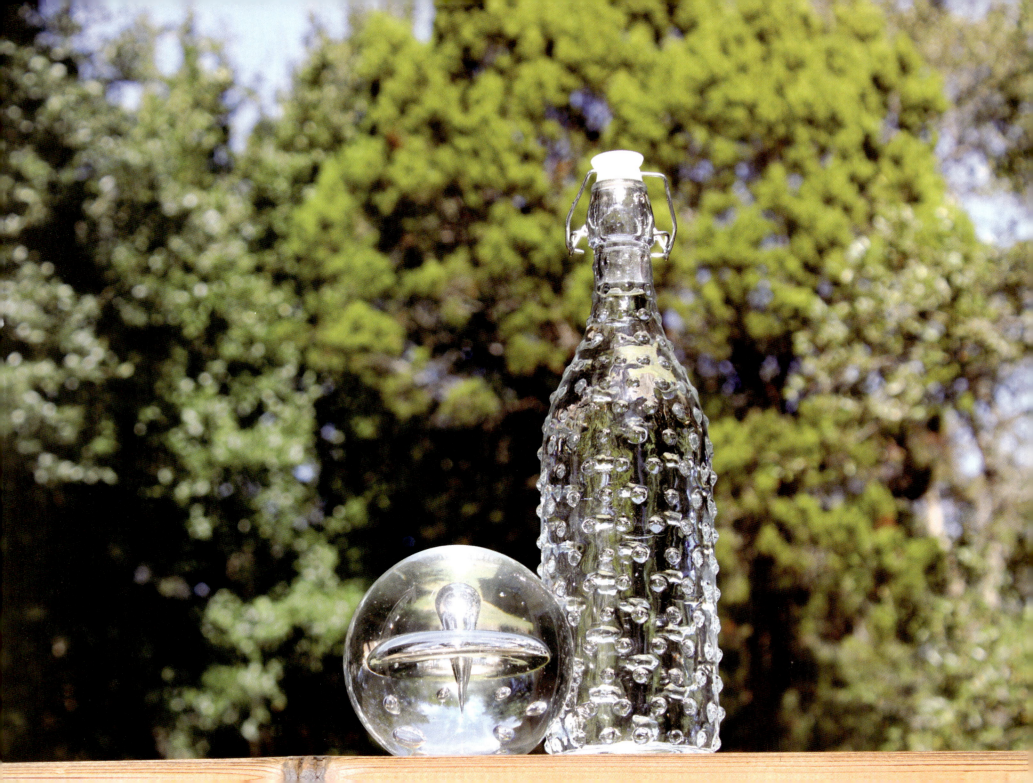

46. Pāṇī (Plain Water)

પાણી

Optimal digestion, body detoxification

- Drink a glass of **WATER** that has been stored in a copper vessel overnight for 8 hours. Drink this water first thing in the morning on an empty stomach (before brushing your teeth) while sitting on the floor in a comfortable cross-legged position

- Avoid consuming water with meals

- Wait at least <u>30 minutes</u> to drink water after each meal

- Wait at least 30 minutes after a meal to take a shower or exercise

- After drinking water wait at least 30 minutes to eat food

- Drink 8+ glasses of water a day - room temperature or lukewarm (avoid cold water)

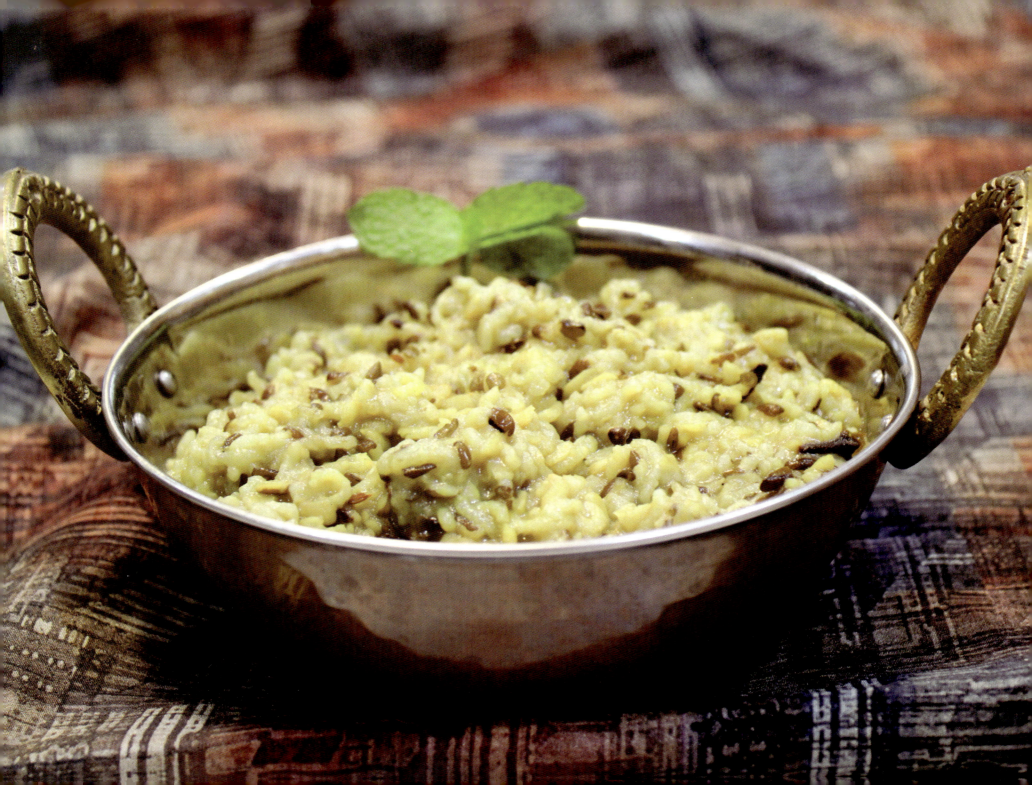

47. Fōtrāvāḷī Dāḷnī Khīchaḍī (Moong Dal Khichdi)

ફોતરાવાળી દાળની ખીચડી

FOR EASY DIGESTION

- Put ½ cup **RICE** and ½ cup **SPLIT MOONG BEANS** in a bowl

- Wash in water at least 3-4 times and let mixture soak for 30 minutes

- In a small pressure cooker heat on low flame ¼ teaspoon of **GHEE** and ¼ cup of **WATER**

- Add ⅛ teaspoon **ORGANIC TURMERIC POWDER**, ¼ teaspoon of **AJWAIN SEEDS**, 1 small **CINNAMON STICK**, 2 **CLOVES**, **SALT** to taste

- Add soaked rice and moong beans in the cooker

- Mix well, close lid of pressure cooker and cook for 3 whistles on medium flame

- Remove from heat and <u>allow pressure to naturally release</u> before opening the lid

- Mix gently and pour a teaspoon of ghee on top to enhance the flavor

- Serve this comfort food in a plate or bowl. Enjoy while hot with **YOGURT** of your choice or with roasted **PAPADUM**

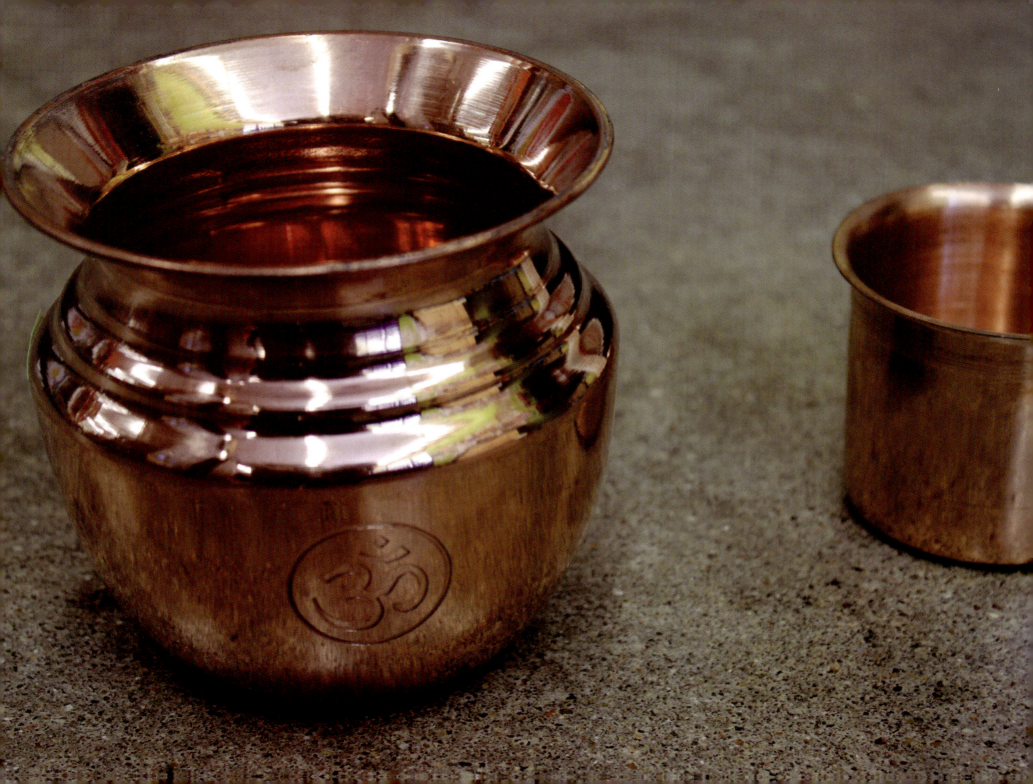

48. Tāmbānō Lōṭō (Water from Copper Vessel)

તાંબાનો લોટો

CLEANSE AND DETOX STOMACH, HEART HEALTHY, AIDS WEIGHT LOSS

- Store **WATER** in an authentic ayurvedic **COPPER VESSEL**, cover with a lid and let it sit overnight at room temperature

- Drink water from the copper vessel <u>first thing</u> in the morning while sitting on the floor in a comfortable cross-legged position

- Wash the copper vessel thoroughly after each use with lemon, salt and water (squeeze juice from ½ lemon into the vessel and mix with ½ cup of water & ½ teaspoon of salt. Shake this solution well for 15-20 seconds to thoroughly clean then rinse with warm water. Dry completely with a clean soft cloth and store in a dry place)

- Repeat daily

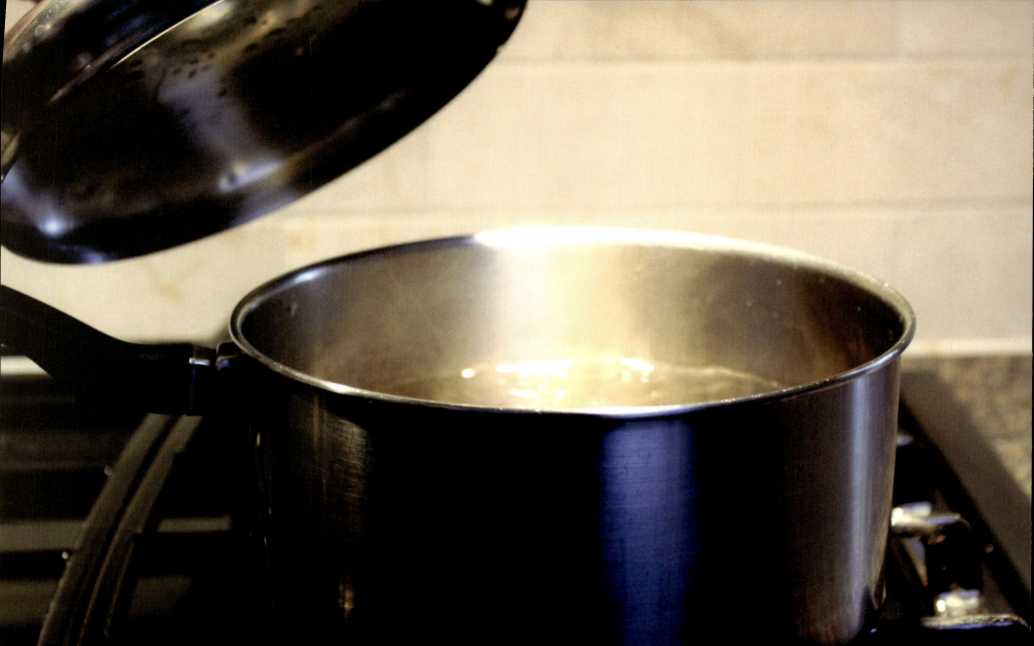

49. Nās (Soothing Steam Facial Inhaler)

નાસ

USEFUL FOR DRY NOSE, CLOGGED SINUSES, CONGESTION, COUGH & UNCLOGS PORES

- Heat 2 cups of **WATER** in a large pot over high heat

- Bring to a boil and turn off the stove

- Drape a towel over your head letting it drop to both sides of your face

- Keeping your <u>eyes closed</u>, lean over and place your face over the steaming pot so you can feel the steam (not to a burning feeling) and still able to breathe

- Inhale the **STEAM** from the pot for as long as you can handle the heat, or a maximum of 5-10 minutes

- Breathe deeply through your nose and mouth

- Blow your nose gently when you finish

- Avoid exposure to cold environment for 30 minutes after steam

- Repeat 2 times a day ideally before bedtime and in the morning as needed

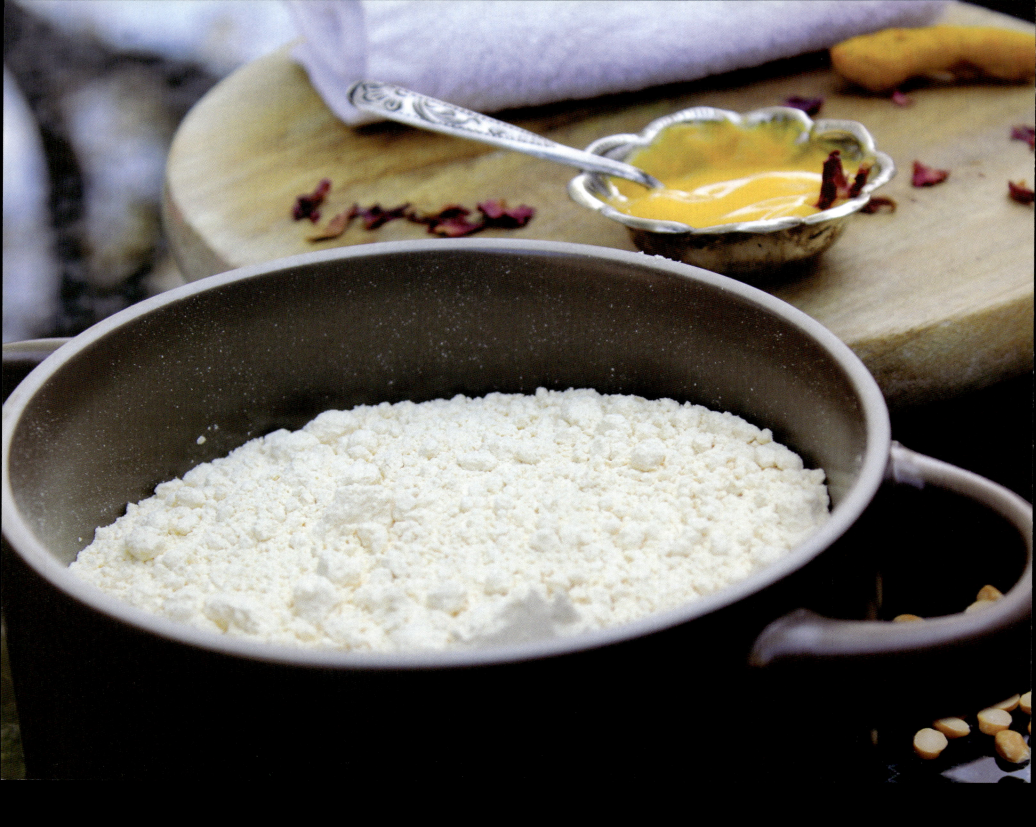

50. Bēsan anē Dahī (Gram Flour Curd Face Mask)
બેસન અને દહી

SKIN MOISTURIZER, EXFOLIATION, CLEANSER, HEALS DRY SKIN

- Wash your hands
- Add 2 tablespoons of **GRAM FLOUR**, 2 teaspoons of **YOGURT** of your choice and ½ teaspoon of **ORGANIC TURMERIC POWDER** in a bowl
- Mix it well to create a smooth thick paste-like consistency
- Apply face mask paste as an even layer on your face (forehead, under eyes, cheeks, on top of nose, below nose, under chin). Note: this can be applied to scrub entire body using more water and flour
- Rub gently in circular motions when applying to the face
- Leave face mask paste on for 15 minutes
- Rinse with water and pat your skin dry
- Repeat twice a week

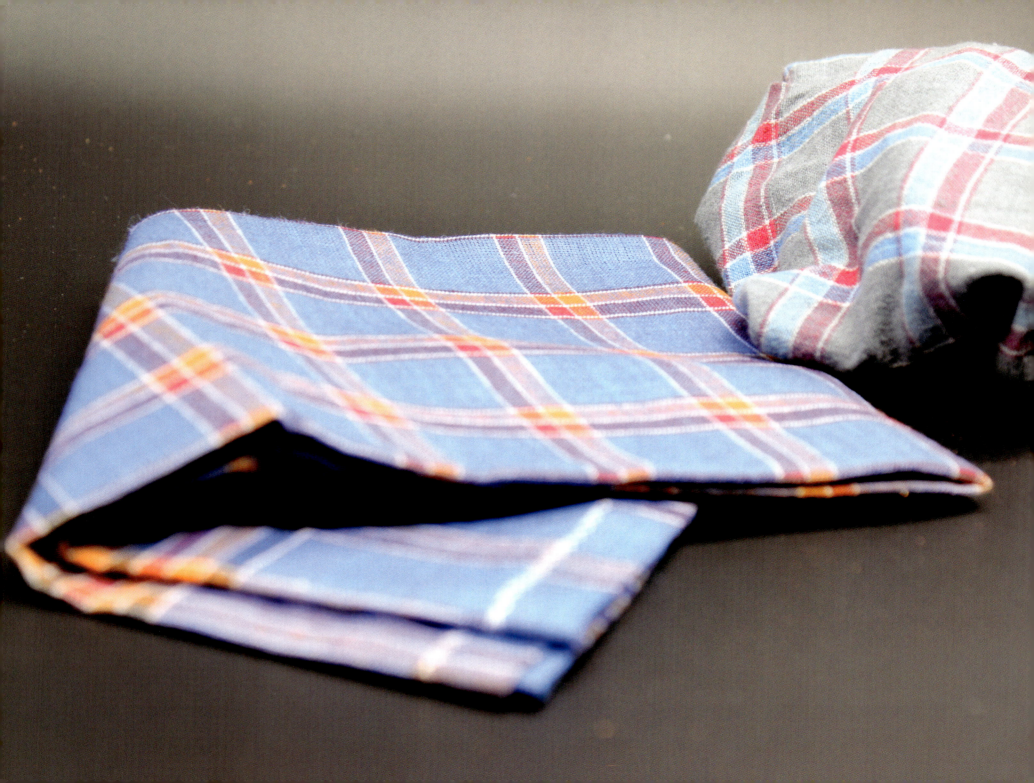

51. Garam Śhēk (Warm Compress)

ગરમ શેક

USEFUL TO RELIEVE EAR INFECTION

- Fold two cotton **HANDKERCHIEF** into medium-sized balls

- Heat a pan on a low flame

- Use one hand to warm a handkerchief on the pan

- Lift away and lightly touch the handkerchief on the other hand. It should be warm enough that your skin can handle without any discomfort or burning

- Apply the warm compress <u>directly over the affected ear for 10-15 seconds</u>

- Use your other hand to warm the second handkerchief on the pan. When warm, alternate the handkerchiefs to cover the affected ear with the warmer handkerchief and maintain heat

- Continue this process for 10-15 minutes

- Turn off the heat

- Repeat 3 times a day as needed

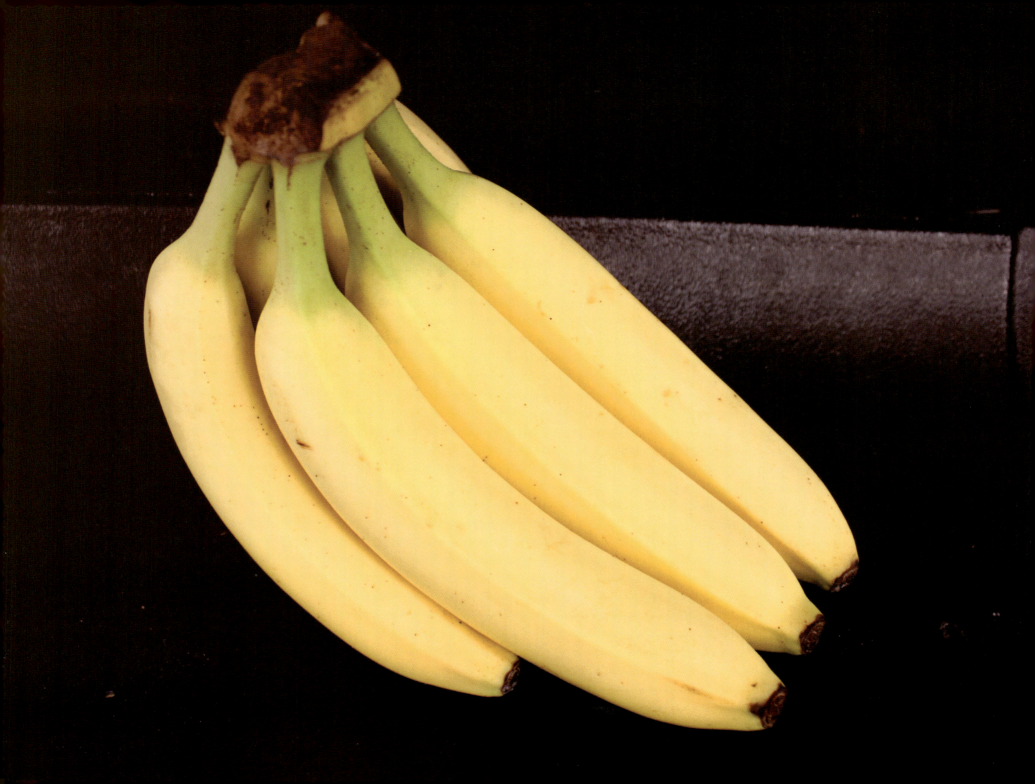

52. Kēḷu (Energy Booster Banana)

కెళు

TO BOOST ENERGY LEVEL, PROVIDES INSTANT ENERGY

- Eat 1 ripe **BANANA** <u>in the morning</u> before, after or with breakfast (not over-ripe banana)

- Repeat daily

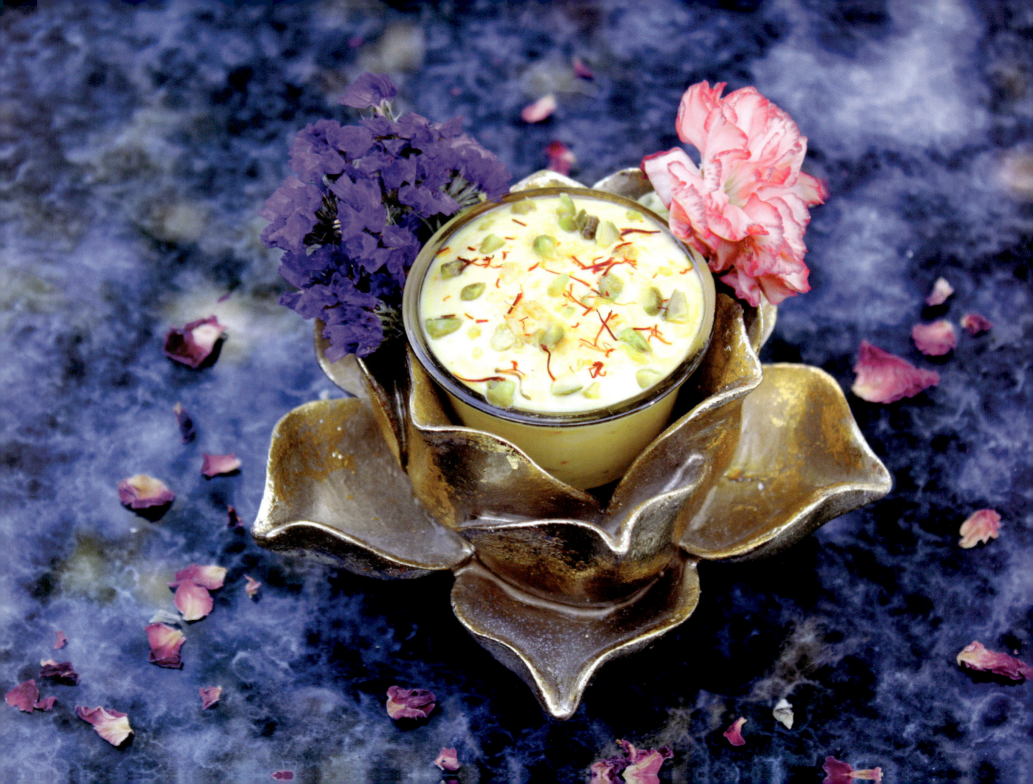

53. Kēsarnu Śhrīkhaṇḍ (Saffron-Infused Yogurt)
કેસરનું શ્રીખંડ

VISUAL ACUITY, AIDS IN MACULAR DEGENERATION, SENSITIVITY TO LIGHT

- Heat 2 teaspoons of **MILK** of your choice in a small pan
- Crush 8 threads of **SAFFRON** to a powder state using your fingers and add to in pan
- Remove pan from the heat and let saffron soak in the milk for 2-3 minutes
- Transfer ½ - 1 cup **PLAIN YOGURT** of your choice to a mixing bowl
- Add 2-3 teaspoons of **SUGAR** of your choice (adjust quantity as per your taste), a pinch of **CARDAMON POWDER** and saffron milk
- Gently whisk and fold the ingredients into the yogurt using a spatula until combined evenly and smooth at the top
- Chill saffron yogurt (also known as *shrikhand*) in the refrigerator for 1-2 hours to thicken before serving
- Scoop into a serving bowl and garnish with a pinch of saffron (optional: chop 3-4 **PISTACHIOS** to small pieces and garnish on top)
- Enjoy this silky smooth, aromatic, flavorful, creamy and heavenly delicacy
- Repeat once a week as needed

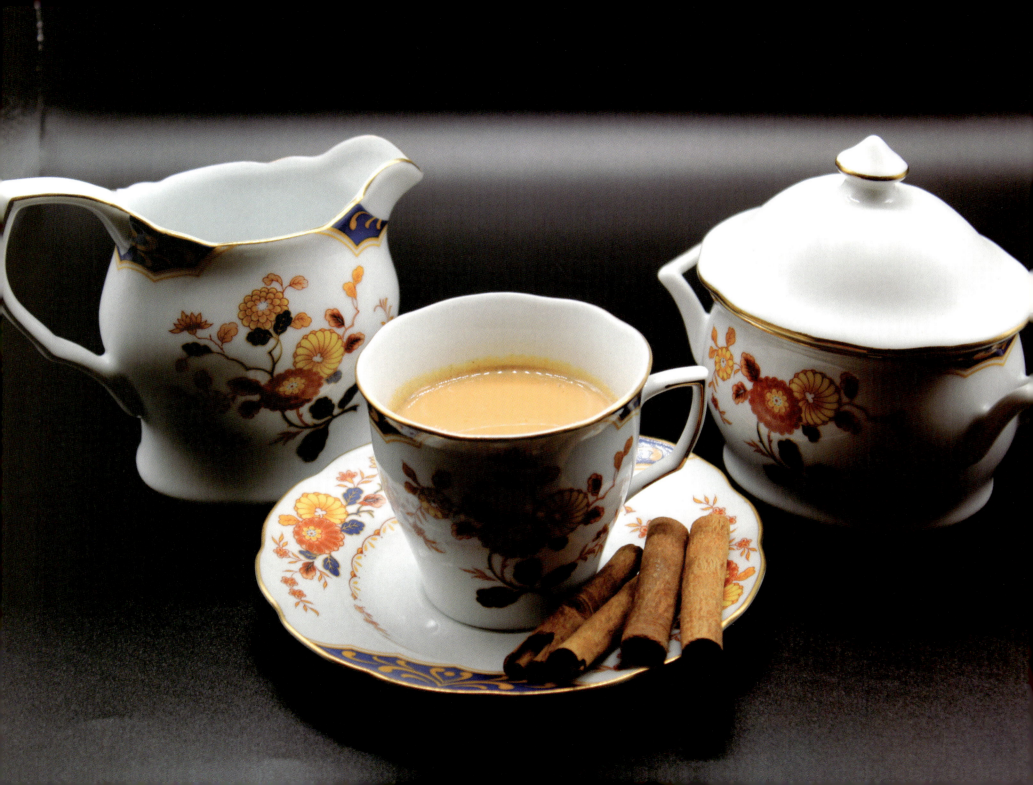

54. Masālā Chā (Aromatic Chai Gujarati Style)
મસાલા ચા

Drives away fatigue

- Combine ½ cup of **MILK** of your choice with ¾ cup cold **WATER** in a pot at medium heat (change ratio of milk and water to your taste)

- Add ¼ teaspoon of **CHAI MASALA POWDER** (homemade or store bought is fine)

- Add 1 teaspoon of your preferred **SUGAR** (optional)

- Add 1 sprig of washed fresh **MINT LEAVES**

- Add ½ inch of freshly grated peeled **GINGER** cut into thin slices

- Add ¼ teaspoon of **CARDAMON SEEDS POWDER**

- Mix and let it simmer gently for 10 minutes to allow the spices to infuse

- Add 1 teaspoon of loose Indian **BLACK TEA** (or 1 tea bag) and let it infuse and steep for few minutes

- Bring the chai to a boil then to a simmer (gently bubbling and rising to top of pot)

- At this point immediately turn off the heat and strain the chai into a teapot or teacup

- Sit back, relax and enjoy drinking this aromatic spicy beverage while hot

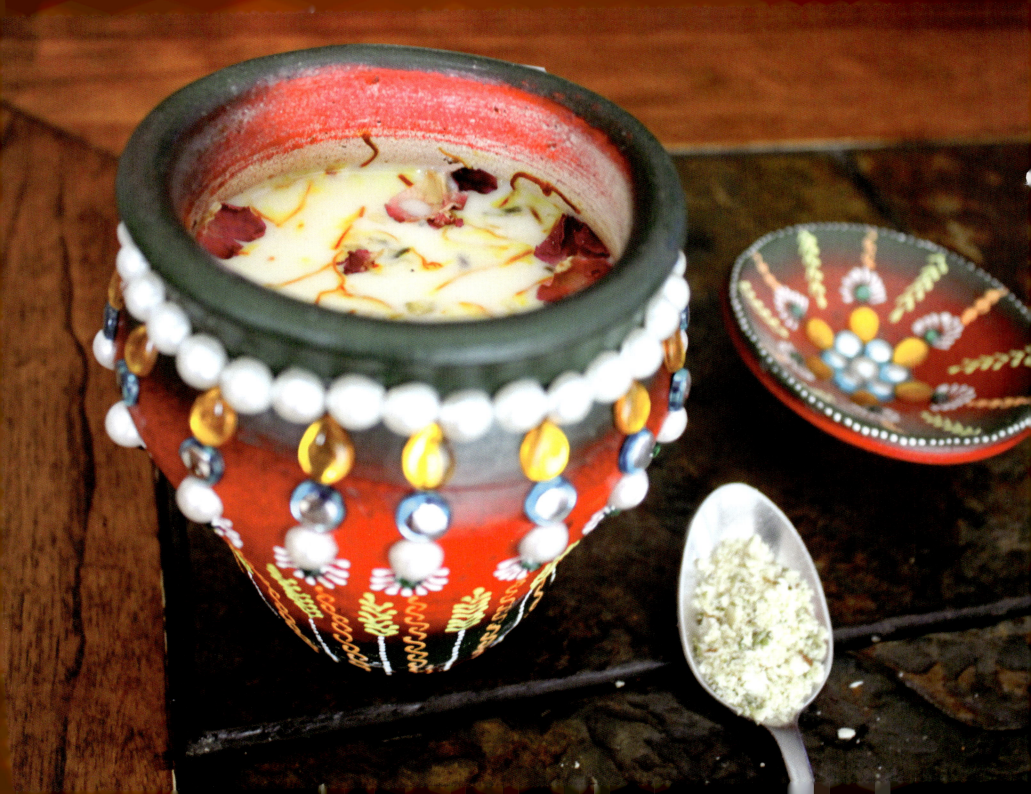

55. Thaṇḍāi (Aromatic Spiced Frappe Shake)
ธรเย

INSTANT ENERGIZER, IMMUNITY BOOST AND BODY DETOX

- Boil 1½ cups **MILK** of your choice in a pot
- Crush 2 tablespoons of **ROCK SUGAR** and mix in pot until the sugar dissolves
- After milk cools down, mix 3 tablespoons of **THANDAI POWDER** (homemade or store bought is fine), stir well and transfer to a large jug
- Garnish with 2 tablespoons of **CRUSHED ALMONDS**, 2 tablespoons of crushed **CASHEW NUTS** and 2-3 **SAFFRON THREADS**
- Mix well and refrigerate this mixture for 2-3 hours
- Pour in a tall glass and indulge in this delicious, cooling frappe as a chilled, refreshing beverage. Keep remaining frappe chilled in the refrigerator for additional servings
- Repeat as needed

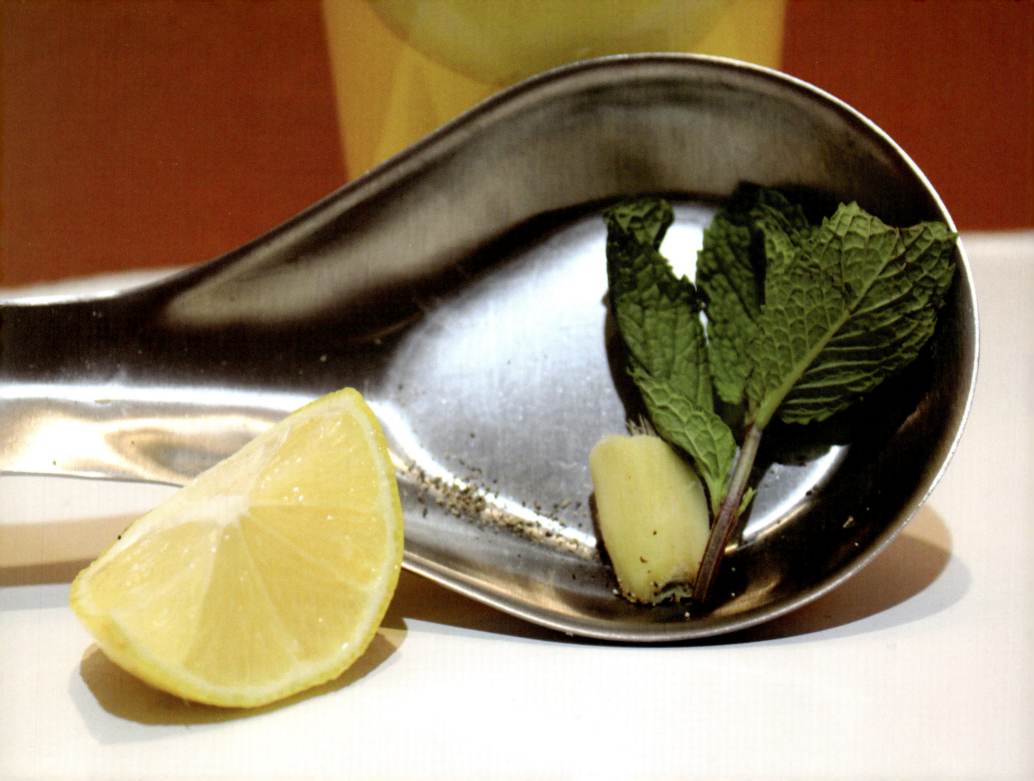

56. Āadu Fudīnānō Ukāḷō (Ginger Mint Shot)

આદુ ફુદીનાનો ઉકાળો

To reduce fever

- Heat ¼ teaspoon **PURE ORGANIC GHEE** in a small pot at medium heat
- Add 1½ glasses of **WATER**
- Sprinkle ¼ teaspoon of **DRY GINGER POWDER** (or squeeze juice out from a ½ inch peeled, shredded fresh **GINGER**)
- Add ¼ teaspoon of **GROUND BLACK PEPPER POWDER**
- Add ¼ teaspoon of **AJWAIN SEEDS**
- Add ¼ teaspoon of **CINNAMON POWDER**
- Add 1 sprig of fresh **MINT LEAVES**
- Let it come to a boil to ½ the size then remove the pot from heat
- Squeeze ¼ fresh **LEMON** in the pot and a pinch of **ORGANIC JAGGERY**
- Mix and pour into a glass
- Enjoy this drink while hot

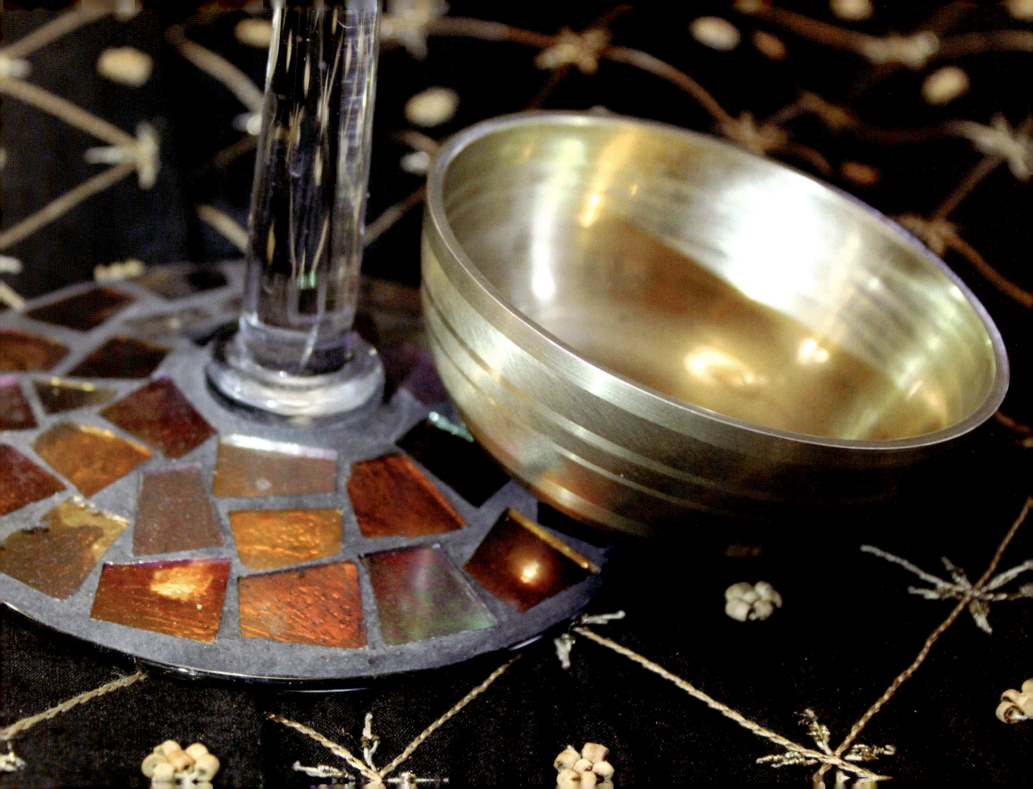

57. Kānsānī Vāḍkī (Ayurvedic Foot Massage)

કાંસાની વાડકી

TO REDUCE FEVER

- Wash your hands

- Heat 1 teaspoon of **CASTOR OIL** to tolerable heat

- Rub the heated oil on the bottom of a **COPPER ZINC TIN METAL BOWL** (also known as *kansani vadki*)

- Bring the well-oiled bowl in contact with the <u>heel of any foot</u> and massage with synchronous circular motions and strokes for 10 minutes

- Repeat on heel of other foot

- Continue every 3-4 hours as needed to balance body temperature

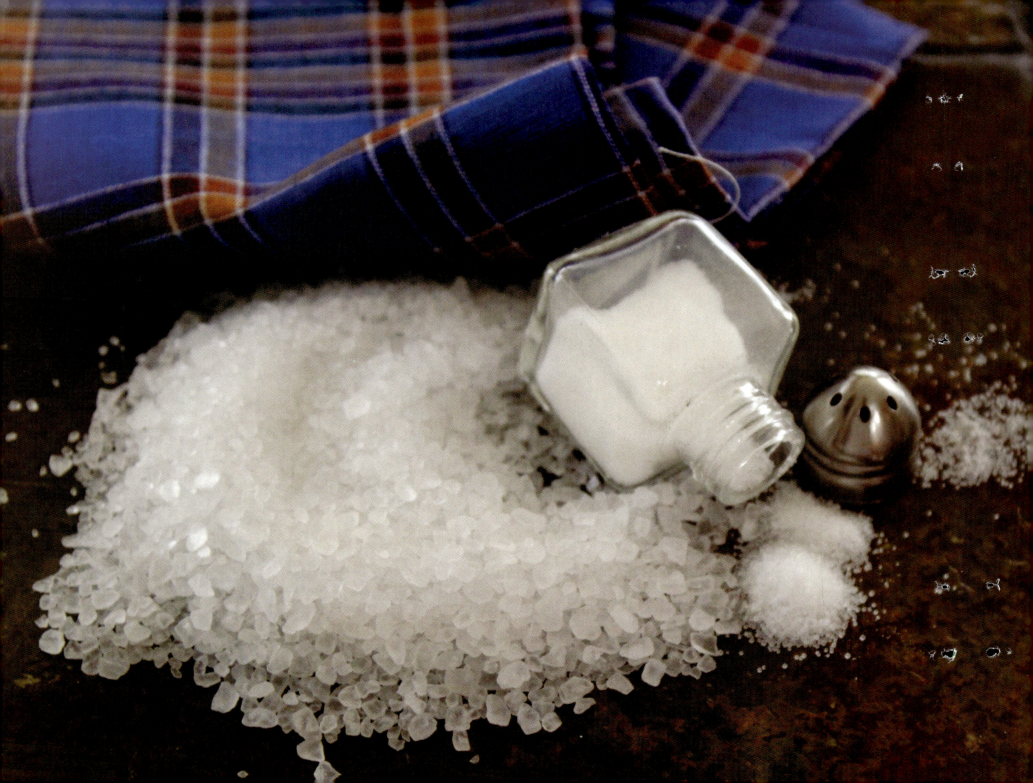

58. Mīṭhānā Pāṇīna Potā (Salt Water Sponge)

મીઠાના પાણીના પોતા

To reduce fever from 101-105 to 98.5 in children

- Fill one pot with **ICE COLD WATER** and **SALT**

- Fill another pot with ice cold water

- Dip handkerchief into pot with ice cold salt water and squeeze water out

- Apply damp handkerchief to forehead (and in parallel, be sure to keep another handkerchief ready which has been dipped in pot with ice cold salt and water squeezed out)

- As you feel the heat drawing out from the forehead the handkerchief will absorb the heat and get warm

- Immediately place first handkerchief into pot with ice cold water, squeeze out the heat and simultaneously put second handkerchief on the forehead

- Continue this process for 30 minutes and measure the temperature

- Repeat for 1-2 hours or until body temperature comes down to normal

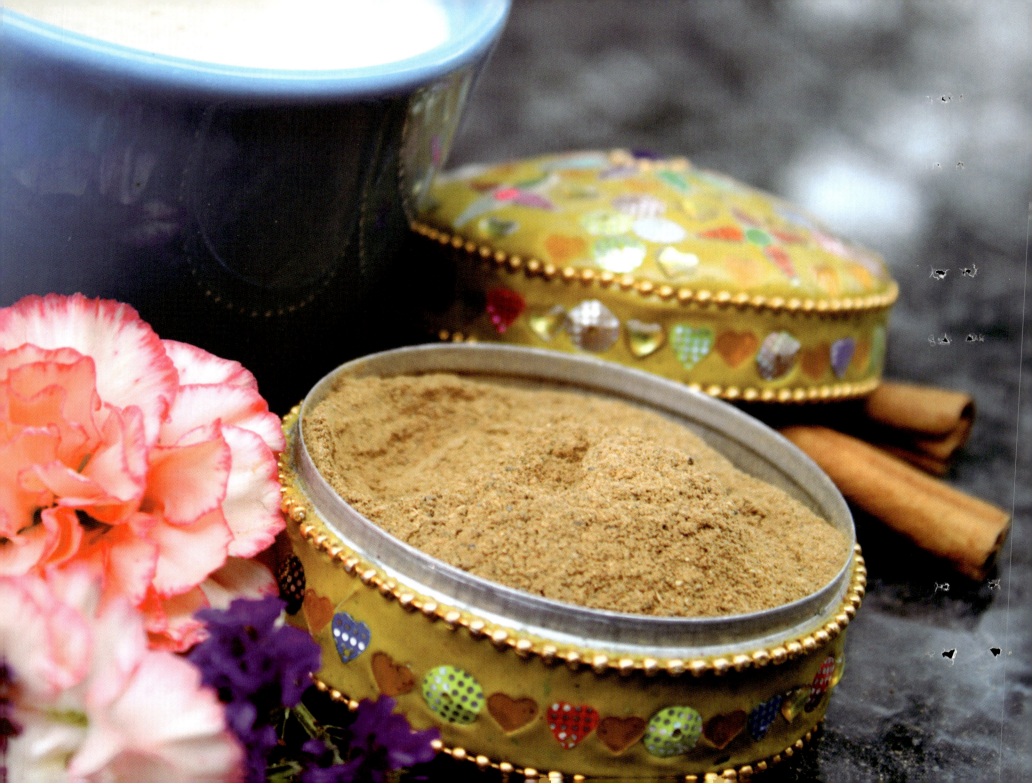

59. Ukāḷō (Spiced Shot)

ઉકાળો

To reduce body temperature

- Add ½ cup **MILK** of your choice to a small pot on a low flame

- Add ½ cup **WATER**

- Add ½ teaspoon of **CHAI MASALA POWDER** (homemade or store bought is fine)

- Add 1½ teaspoon of your preferred **SUGAR**

- Add a pinch of **CARDAMOM POWDER**

- <u>Mix well</u> and bring to a boil

- Turn off the heat and pour into a cup

- Enjoy this restorative drink while hot

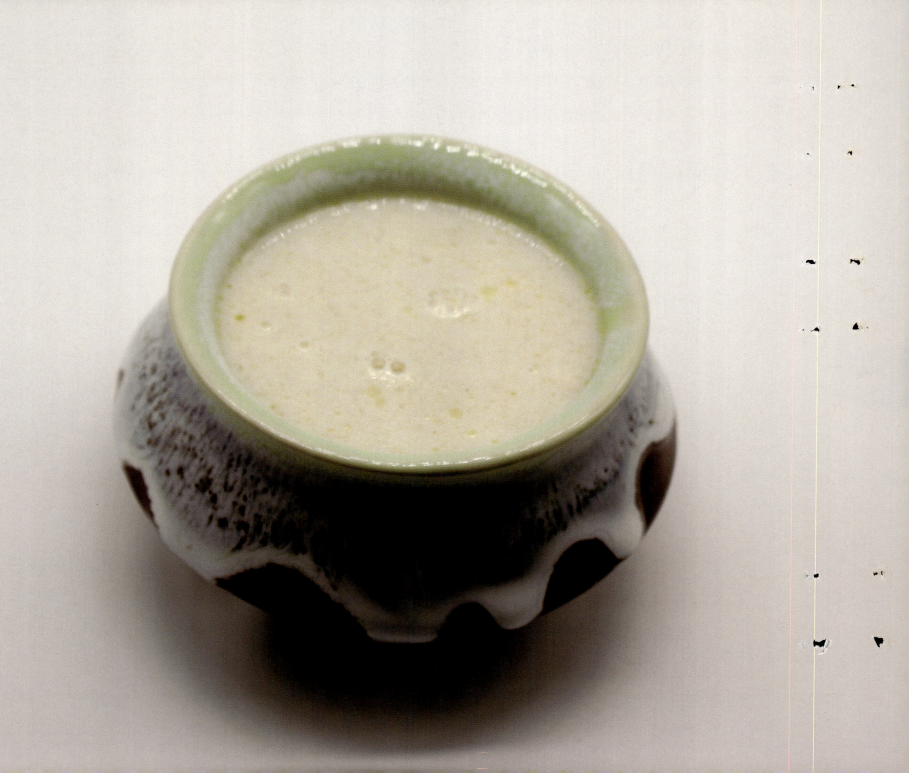

60. Bājrīnō Kāḍhō (Creamy Millet Porridge)

બાજરીનો કાઢો

TO REDUCE BODY FEVER FROM VIRAL INFECTION AND EXHAUSTION

- Heat a small pan on low flame

- Add 1 tablespoon of **PURE ORGANIC GHEE** and let it melt

- Add 1½ tablespoons of fine, organic **MILLET FLOUR** and sauté for 2 minutes

- Pour 1 cup of **MILK** of your choice and stir continuously so no lumps are formed (alternate option: use ¼ cup hot **WATER** and ¾ cup milk of your choice)

- Let this mixture simmer and boil for 1 minute, then turn off the heat

- Add **SALT** to taste

- Pour into a serving bowl and mix

- Enjoy this porridge while hot

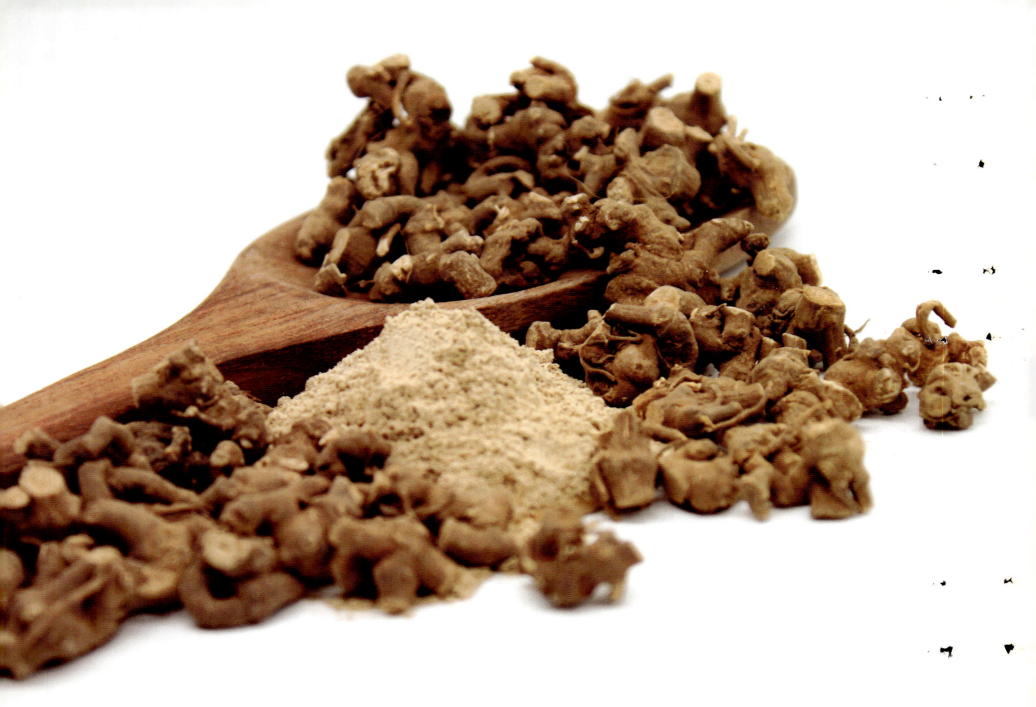

61. Gaṇṭhōḍānō Ukāḷō (Zesty Peepramul Shot)
ગંઠોડાનો ઉકાળો

TO HELP CONTROL COUGH, COLD, FLU

- Rinse pot with water and do not dry the pot
- Add 1 cup **WATER**
- Sprinkle 1 teaspoon **PEEPRAMUL POWDER** in the pot and cover with lid
- Let sit for a few minutes
- Heat over medium flame when water comes to a boil, add 1 teaspoon of **ORGANIC JAGGERY**
- Add ½ teaspoon of **CHAI MASALA POWDER** (homemade or store bought is fine)
- Stir the ingredients and let it boil for 2-3 minutes
- Enjoy this drink while hot

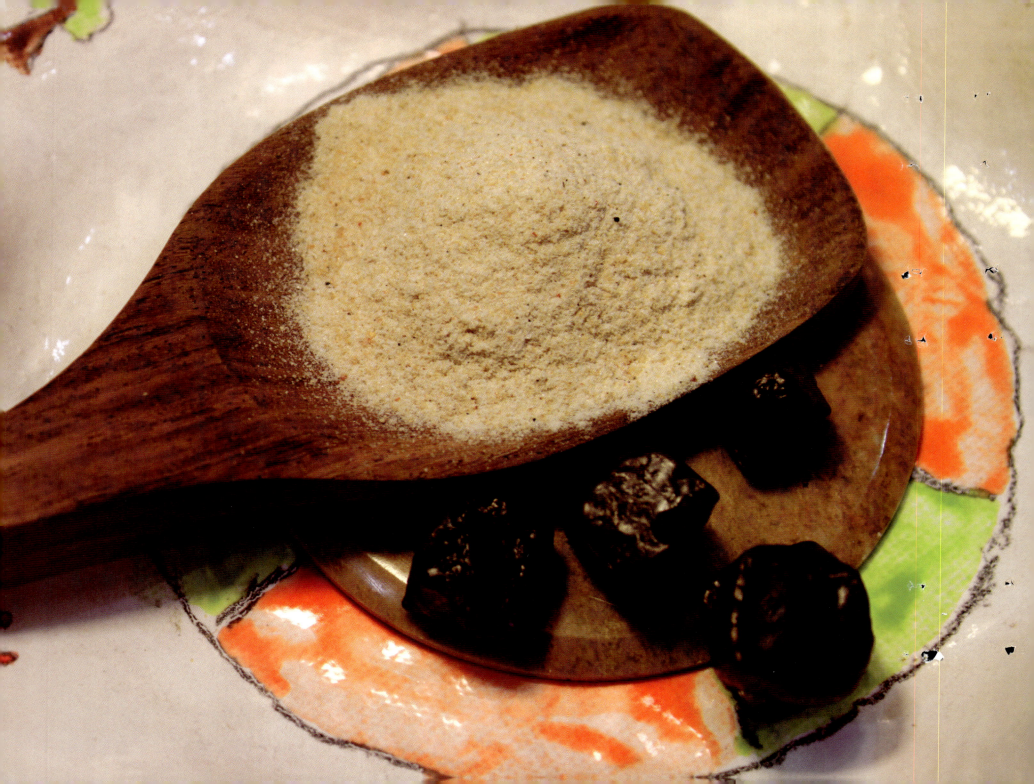

62. Hīṅg Marīnō Ukāḷō (Asafoetida Pepper Shot)

હીંગ મરીનો ઉકાળો

FOR GAS RELIEF, STOMACH PAIN

- Heat ½ teaspoon **PURE ORGANIC GHEE** in a small pot at low temperature

- Add 1½ cups of **WATER**

- Sprinkle ¼ teaspoon of powder **ORGANIC ASAFOETIDA**, ¼ teaspoon of **GROUND BLACK PEPPER POWDER** and a pinch of **SALT**

- After it comes to a boil remove from the heat

- Squeeze 2-3 drops of juice from a fresh **LEMON**

- Mix with a spoon and pour into a mug

- Enjoy this drink while hot

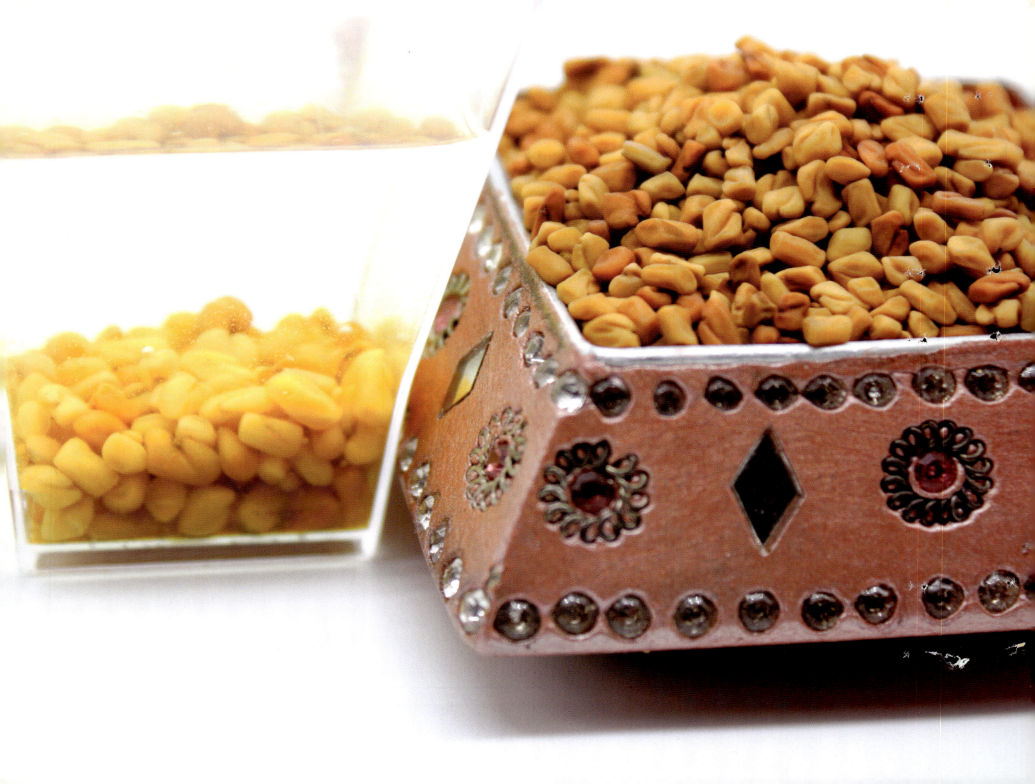

63. Mēthī (Soaked Fenugreek)

મેથી

TO ALLEVIATE GAS/DIARRHEA FOR CHILDREN

- Soak 1 teaspoon of **FENUGREEK SEEDS** in a ½ cup of **WATER** for 6-8 hours
- Filter the water in a bowl and drink it
- Then mix soaked seeds with ¼ teaspoon of **ORGANIC JAGGERY**
- Chew this mixture
- Avoid drinking water for 30 minutes afterward

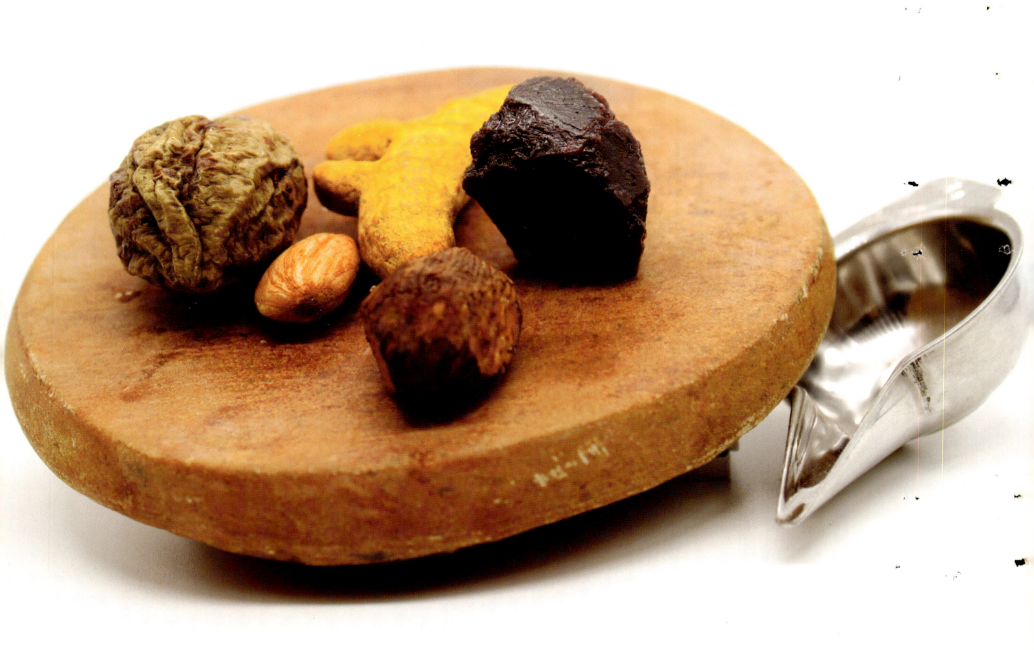

64. Ghasārō (Health Tonic)

ધસારો

PROVIDE GOOD HEALTH AND WHOLESOME LIFE FOR BABIES

- Wash your hands
- Wash flat grinding stone with hot water and let it dry
- Rub these ingredients one at a time on the stone very gently. Repeat daily for new born baby from 15th day until the baby is 1 year
  - Every day total 1 stroke for **DRIED TUMERIC ROOT**, 1 stroke for **FRESH WHOLE NUTMEG**, 1 stroke for **RAW ORGANIC ALMOND**
  - On alternate days also include 2 strokes for **HARDE**
  - Once a week also include 2 strokes for **SANCHAL** (Indian black rock salt)
- Use your finger to collect what is left on the stone onto a clean, sterile spoon
- Mix ⅛ teaspoon **ORGANIC HONEY** using your finger
- Immediately give this fresh health tonic to the baby to swallow (total ¼ teaspoon in volume; increase dosage to ½ teaspoon at age 3 months)
- Wash and <u>dry the ingredients after each use</u>

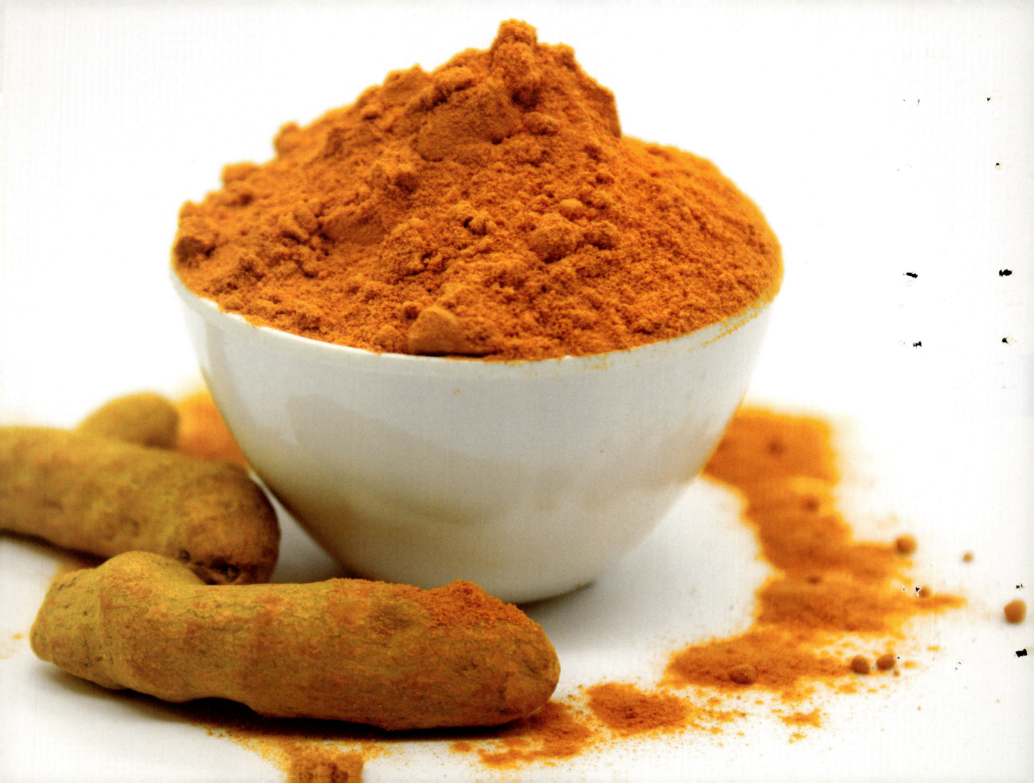

65. Haḷdar Chōpaḍvī (Turmeric Gum Massage)

હળદર ચોપડવી

FOR HEALTHY TEETH AND PROVIDE RELIEF FOR GUMS

- Wash your hands

- Mix 1 teaspoon **GROUND ORGANIC TURMERIC POWDER** with ½ teaspoon of **SALT** and ½ teaspoon of **PURE ORGANIC GHEE** in a small bowl

- Massage <u>gently on gums</u>

- After 5 minutes rinse your mouth with **WATER**

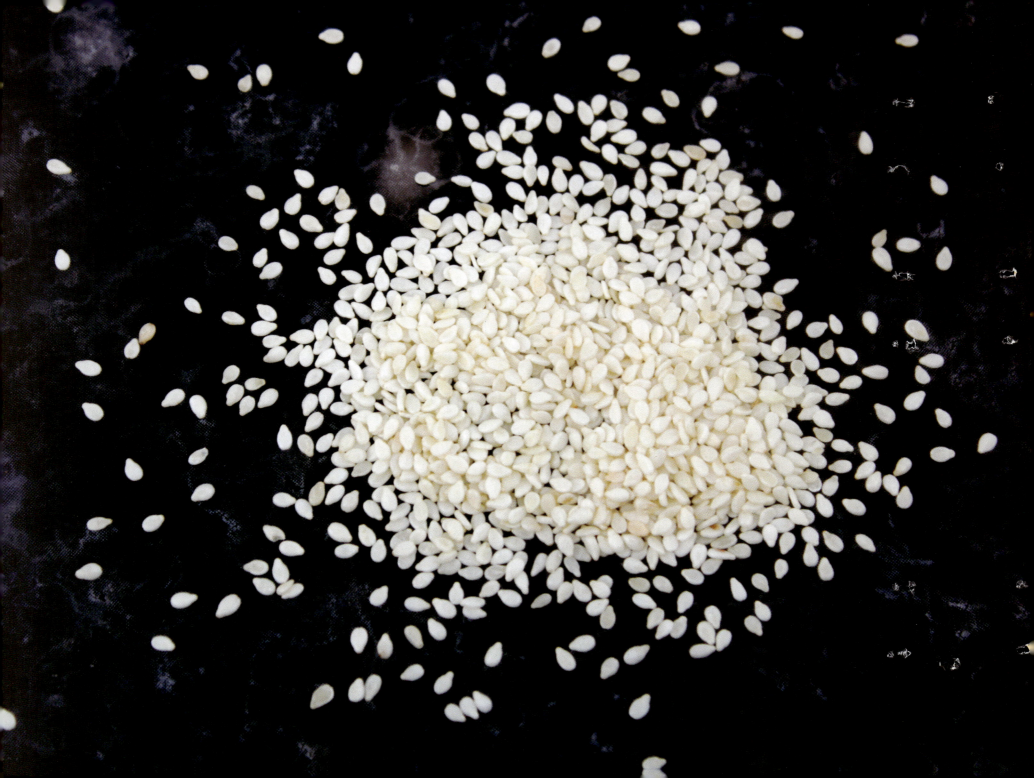

66. Vāaḷ Māṭē Tēl Māliśh (Nourishing Hair Massage)

વાળ માટે તેલ માલિશ

PREVENTS HAIR LOSS, MOISTURIZES HAIR AND SCALP, ENCOURAGES HAIR GROWTH

- Wash your hands
- Pour 2-3 tablespoons of **ORGANIC SESAME OIL** into your hands
- Rub your hands together back and forth to warm the oil
- Beginning with your hairline, use your fingertips to gently massage the oil to the roots, back of your scalp, and continue into the ends of the hair strands
- Continue massaging your hair for 10 minutes and add more oil if needed
- Leave the oil in your hair for at least 2 hours (or overnight)
- Damp a towel with **WATER** and heat in a microwave for 60 seconds or until the towel is hot to touch (alternatively you can heat the towel in running hot water for a few minutes). Be careful it is not too hot to burn the skin. Squeeze out any extra water
- Wrap the hot towel around your head and leave on for 10-15 minutes
- Rinse the oil from your hair with a mild shampoo and cooler water
- Repeat this healing and cooling, essential oil massage treatment 1-2/week as needed

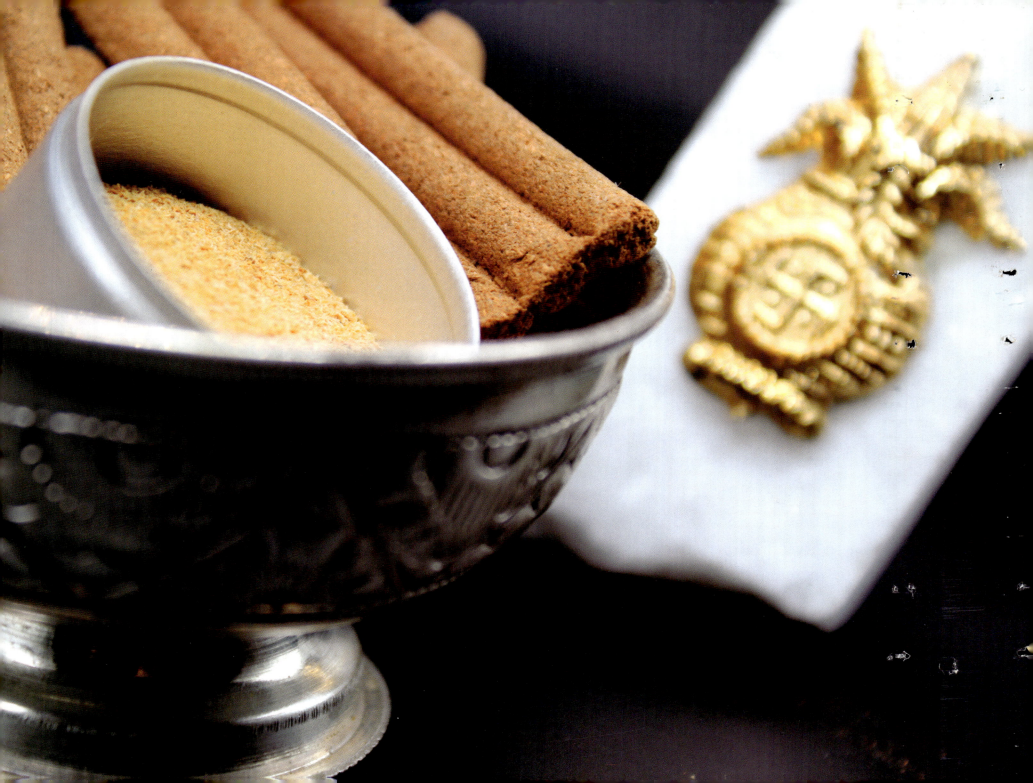

67. Chandan Lagāvō (Sandalwood Creamy Gel Paste)

ચંદન લગાવો

RELIEF FROM HEADACHE

- Mix ¼ teaspoon of **PURE SANDALWOOD POWDER** with a few drops of **WATER** to create a paste-like consistency

- Apply this precious fragrant paste topically on the <u>center of your forehead</u> between the eyebrows

- Repeat daily as needed

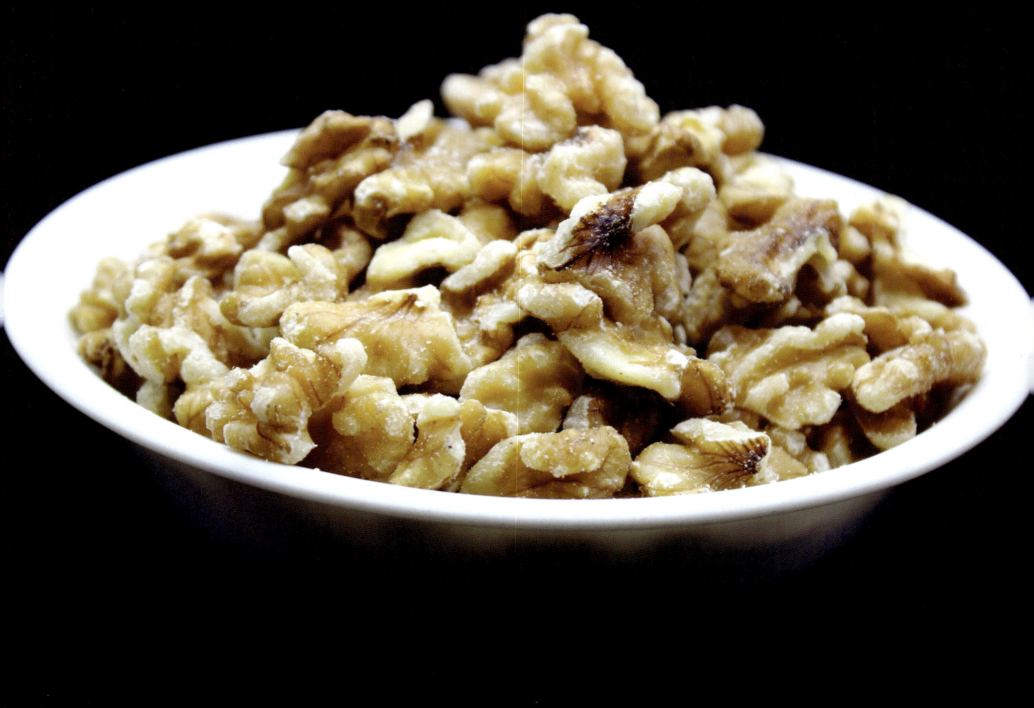

68. Akhrōṭ (Anti-Oxidant Rich Walnuts)
અખરોટ

FOR HEART HEALTHY AND BRAIN HEALTH

- Eat 2 <u>shelled</u> whole **WALNUTS** daily with breakfast (total 4 pieces)

- Take time to chew slowly

- Repeat daily

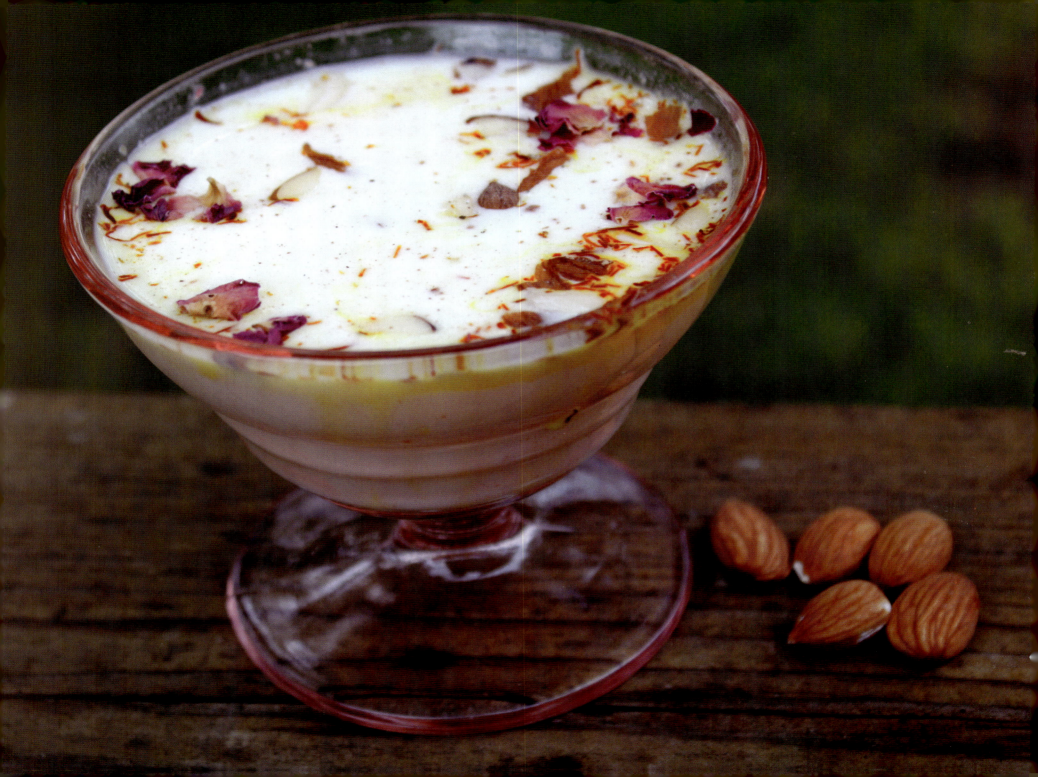

69. Badām Pīstānu Doodh (Spiced Almond Latte)

બદામ પીસ્તાનું દૂધ

TO IMPROVE IMMUNITY, ENERGIZE BODY, BALANCE MIND

- Heat **WATER** in a pot and as soon as the water starts to boil, turn off the heat. Add 7 **ORGANIC WHOLE ALMONDS** to the water and let it sit for few minutes. Then rinse the water, remove the skin and chop the almonds

- Warm 1 cup of **MILK** of your choice in a small pot over medium heat

- When warm, add 2 tablespoons of chopped almonds

- Chop and add 3-5 shelled unsalted **PISTACHIOS**

- Add 1 tablespoon of your preferred **SUGAR**, few grates (or pinch) of fresh **NUTMEG** and ¼ teaspoon of crushed **CARDAMOM POWDER**

- Gently crush 4 threads of **ORGANIC SAFFRON** to a powder state using your fingers, Add to pot and stir these ingredients well

- <u>Simmer for 5 minutes</u> to let the flavors infuse and stir continuously

- Turn off the heat and pour into a glass

- Enjoy this delicious latte sipping hot or as a chilled, refreshing drink

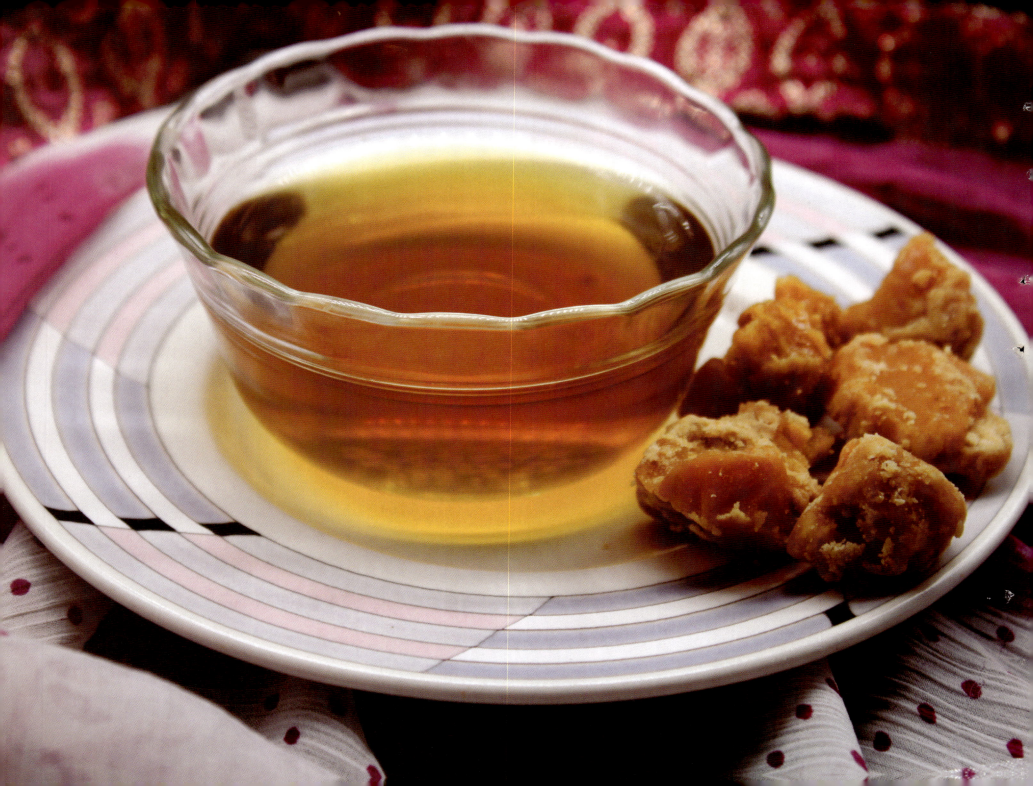

70. Gōḷnu Pāṇī (Blissful Jaggery Drink)

ગોળનું પાણી

FOR IMMUNITY BOOST, AFTER COMPLETION OF A FAST

- Grate 2 tablespoons of **ORGANIC JAGGERY**

- Boil 1 cup of **WATER**, add jaggery in a pot and stir well

- After jaggery melts, add 1 teaspoon of **GHEE** and mix

- Remove pan from the heat and close the lid

- <u>Let it cool for 1 hour</u> then sieve the water

- Pour in a glass and enjoy this blissful drink

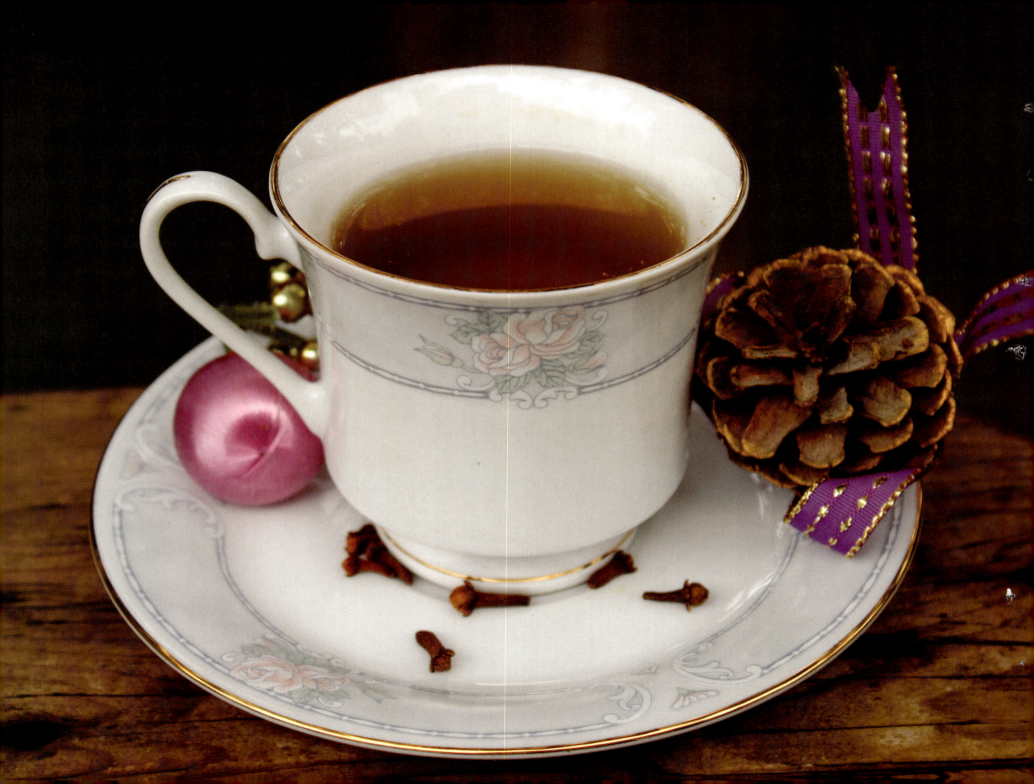

71. Lavīṅgnu Pāṇī (Soothing Clove Tea)

લવીંગનુ પાણી

FOR IMMUNITY BOOST, AFTER COMPLETION OF A FAST

- Crush 2 **ORGANIC CARDAMON PODS**

- Put 1½ cups of **WATER** in a pot on medium flame

- Add 3 whole **CLOVES**, 2 teaspoons of **ROCK SUGAR**, 2 **CINNAMON STICKS** and crushed cardamom in pot

- Boil water mixture til it reduces to ½ half the size

- Let mixture <u>steep for 10 minutes then turn off the heat</u>

- Pour into a serving bowl to let it cool

- After the mixture cools, strain using a metal tea strainer into a cup

- Enjoy this tea while hot

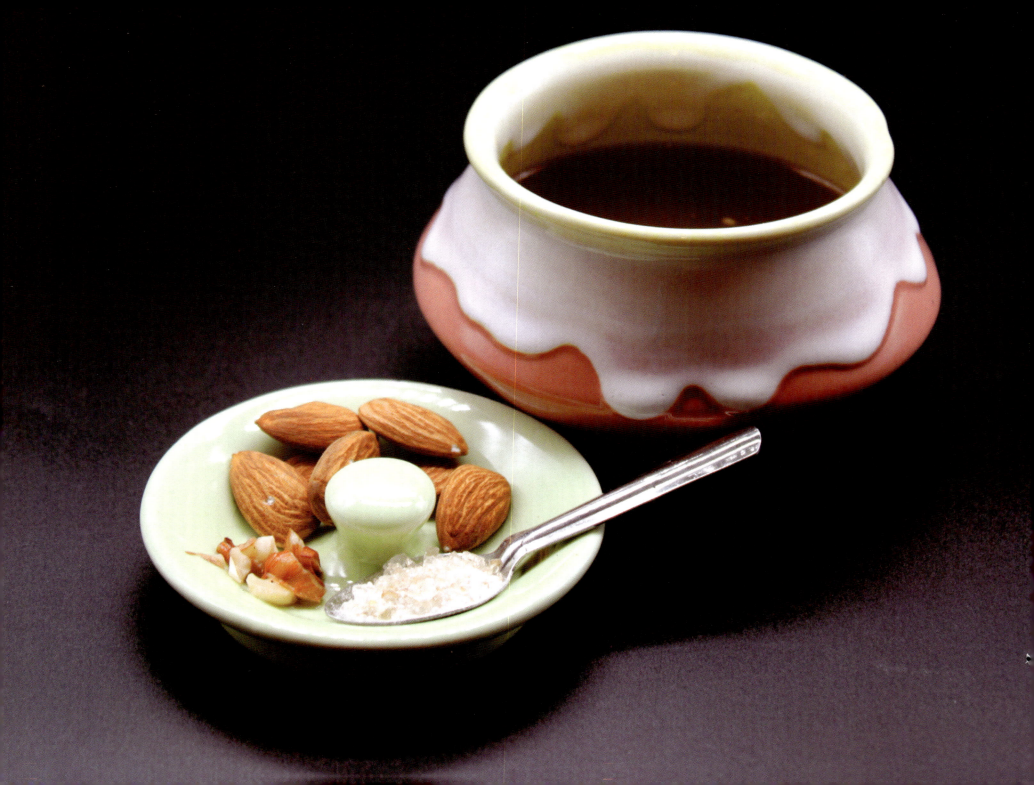

72. Gundarnī Rāab (Edible Gum Almond Porridge)

ગુંદરની રાબ

FOR IMMUNITY BOOST, AFTER COMPLETION OF A FAST, POSTPARTUM HEALING

- Heat 2 tablespoons of **GHEE** in a pan on low flame
- Crush 2 tablespoons of **EDIBLE GUM CRYSTALS** to a fine powder
- Sauté this for 2 minutes (the crystals will bubble and grow in size)
- Add 1 cup of **WATER** and let it boil
- Increase flame to medium-low stirring continuously until the <u>crystals completely dissolve</u> and the mixture thickens (approximately 10 minutes)
- Add 1½ teaspoons **ORGANIC JAGGERY** and mix well until the jaggery melts
- Cut 3 **ORGANIC WHOLE ALMONDS** into fine slivers
- Add slivered almonds, ½ teaspoon of **DRY GINGER POWDER** and ½ teaspoon of **PEEPRAMUL POWDER**
- Stir these ingredients and let it boil 1 minute
- Turn off the stove and transfer to a serving bowl
- Indulge in this healthy, soothing porridge while piping hot

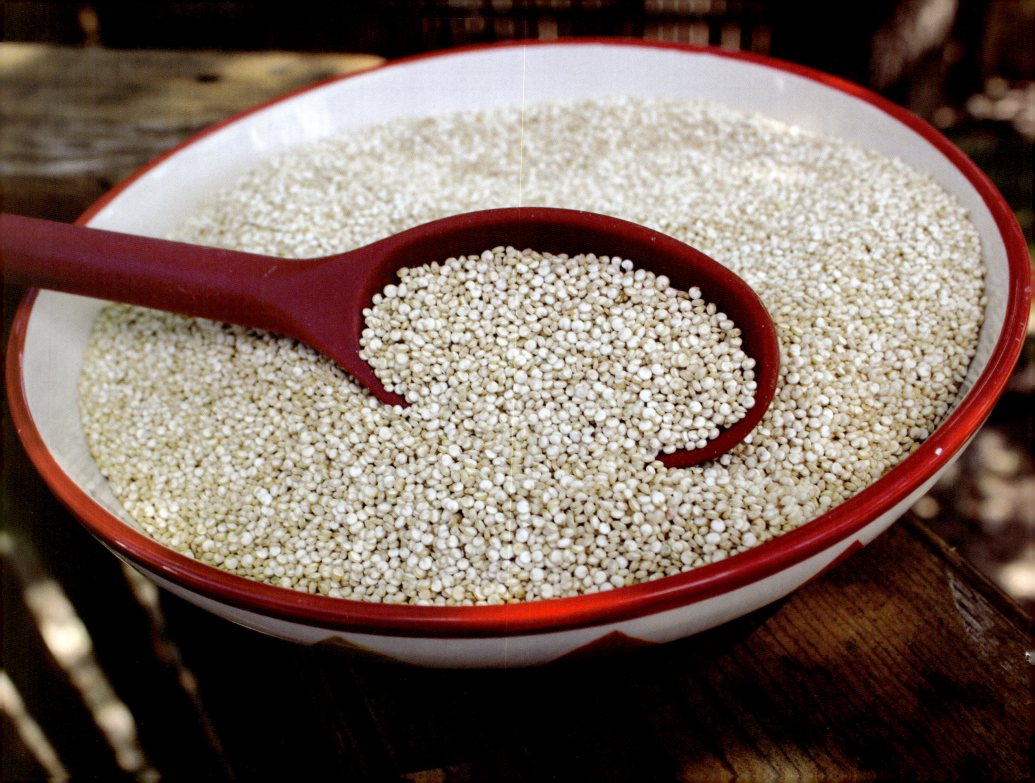

73. KhasKhas (Poppy Seeds Ghee Syrup)

ખસખસ

To Alleviate diarrhea and indigestion

- Heat 1 teaspoon of **GHEE** in a small pot

- When ghee melts, add 1 teaspoon of **POPPY SEEDS**

- Let it <u>roast</u> for 1 minute

- Turn off the stove and let it cool down

- Add ½ teaspoon of roasted seeds in an 8 ounce glass of **WATER**

- Enjoy this syrup

- Repeat 2-3 times a day as needed

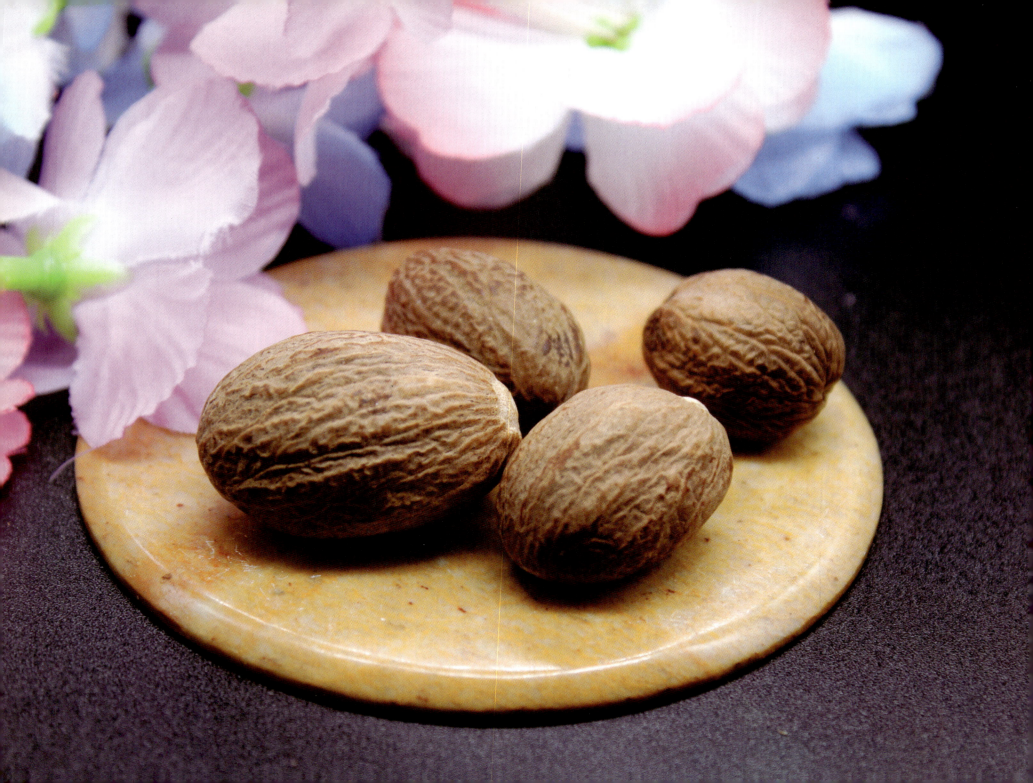

74. Jāiphaḷnu Doodh (Sleepy Nutmeg Elixir)

જાયફળનું દૂધ

FOR SLEEP AID, IMPROVE INSOMNIA AND SLEEP DISORDERS

- Heat 1 cup of **MILK** of your choice in a pan on medium heat

- Add a pinch of **ORGANIC NUTMEG POWDER** (do not exceed ¼ teaspoon as it can cause problems. As always consult your doctor)

- Enjoy this sleepy elixir 1-2 hours before bedtime

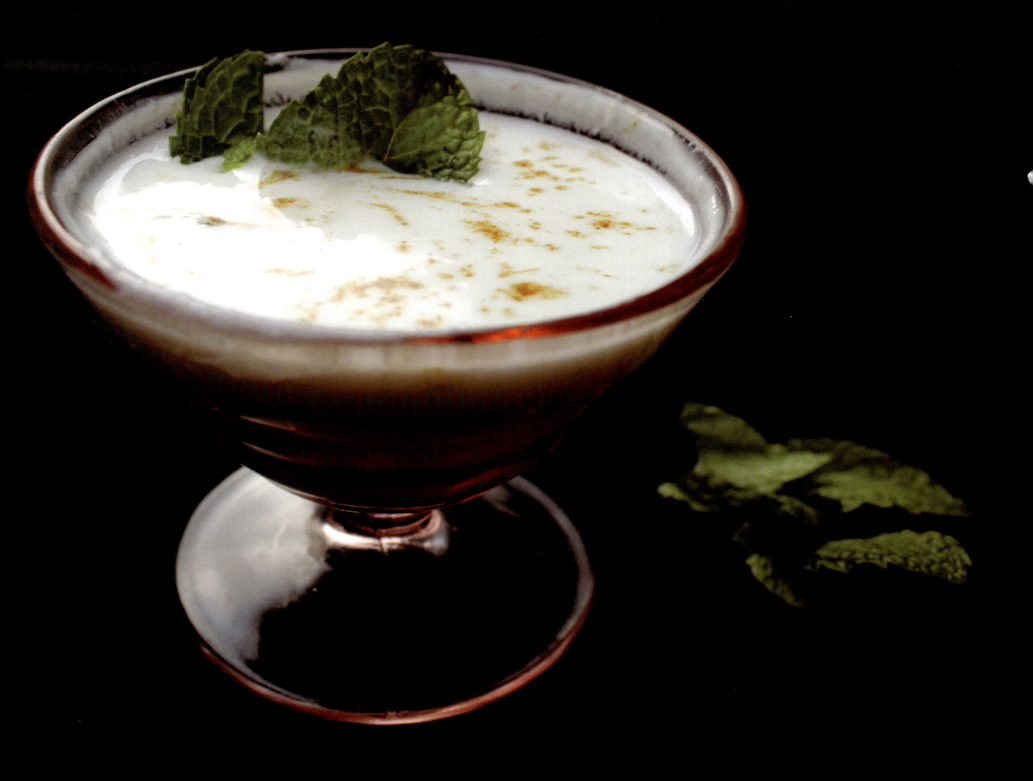

75. Jeerāvāḷi Chhāś (Cumin Spiced Buttermilk)

જીરાવાળી છાશ

TO GET RID OF GAS AND IRRITABLE BOWEL SYNDROME

- In bowl add 1 cup of plain **YOGURT** of your choice

- Roast 1 teaspoon **CUMIN SEEDS** and grind to a fine powder

- Sprinkle roasted powdered cumin seeds and **SALT** to taste to the yogurt

- Whisk it well til no lumps

- Add 2 cups of chilled **WATER** to thin the yogurt

- Whisk it well again

- Pour in a glass

- Enjoy this savory drink <u>after a meal</u> (refrigerate extra)

- This can be served garnished with 1 sprig of chopped **MINT** and ½ sprig of chopped **CILANTRO**

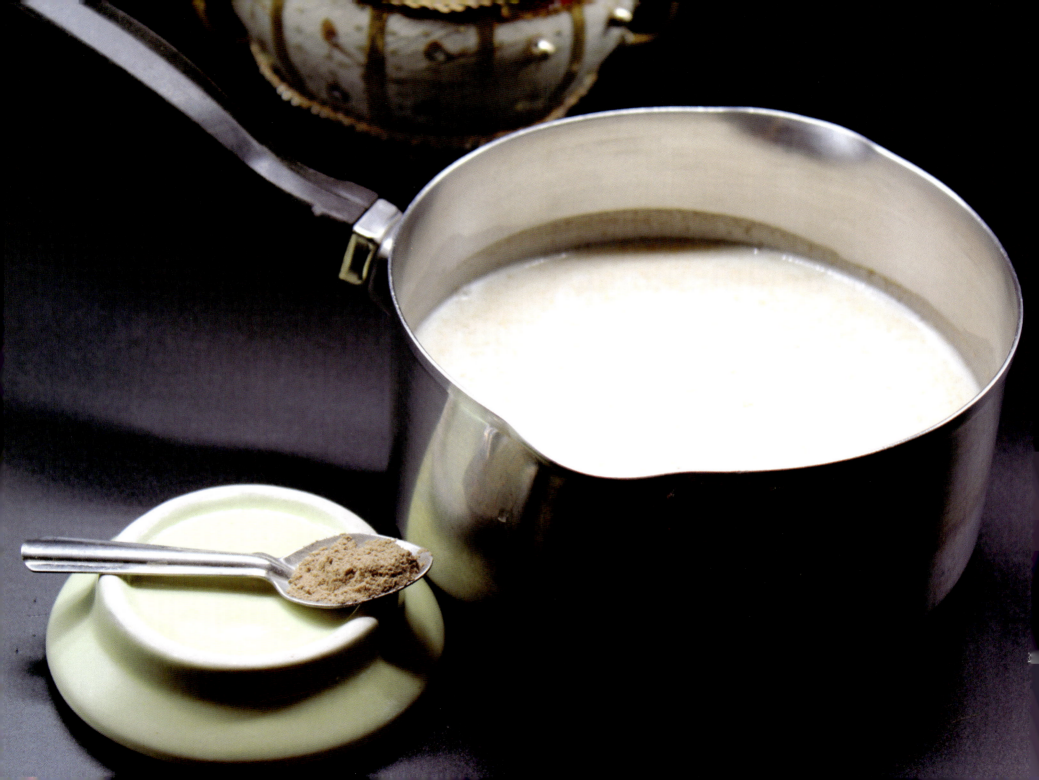

76. Soonth Pipramulnu Doodh (Ginger Peepramul Latte)

સૂંઠ પીપરામૂળનું દૂધ

REDUCES JOINT PAIN

- Rinse pot with water and do not dry the pot

- Add 1 cup **MILK** of your choice

- Sprinkle ½ teaspoon **GINGER POWDER** and 1 teaspoon **PEEPRAMUL POWDER** in the pot and cover with lid

- Let sit for 3-5 minutes to allow the powders to settle down

- Heat over medium flame and stir continuously

- When the milk comes to a boil turn off the flame

- Pour in a mug and enjoy this latte while hot

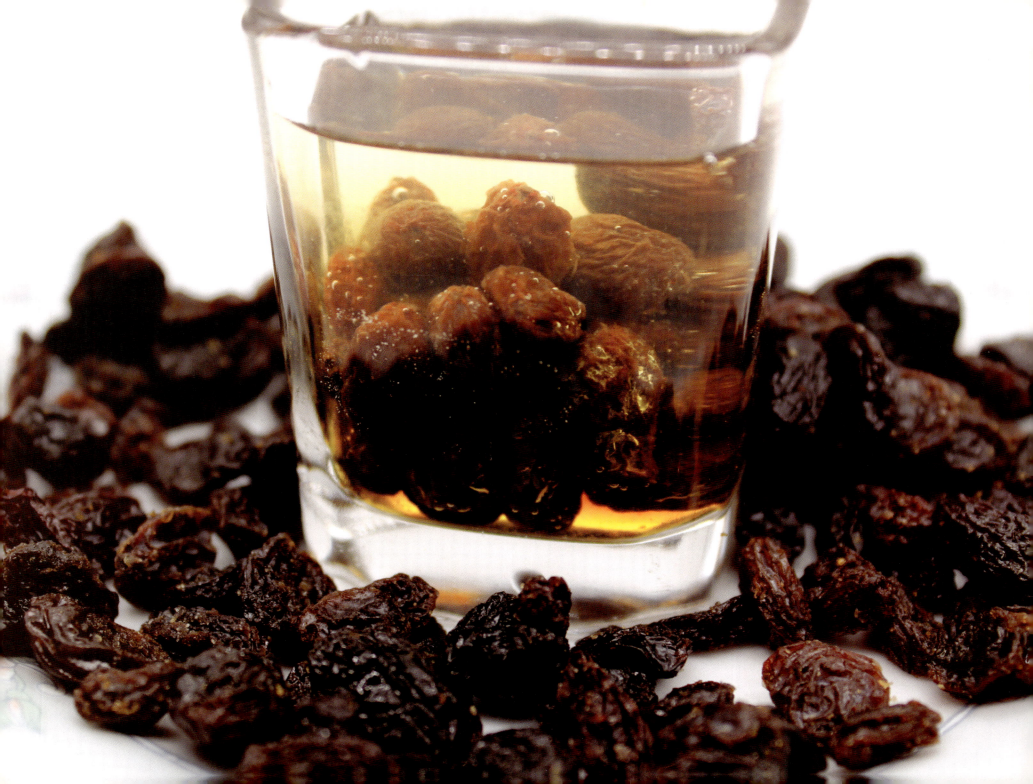

77. Kāḷī Drākṣh (Tasty Soaked Black Raisins)

કાળી દ્રાક્ષ

REGULATES BLOOD PRESSURE LEVEL, BLOOD PURIFIER, IMPROVES HEMOGLOBIN LEVEL

- Soak 10 **BLACK RAISINS** <u>overnight</u> in a 4 ounce glass of **WATER** and cover with a lid

- In the morning strain the water to a small bowl and eat the raisins on an empty stomach

- Drink the strained water

- Repeat daily

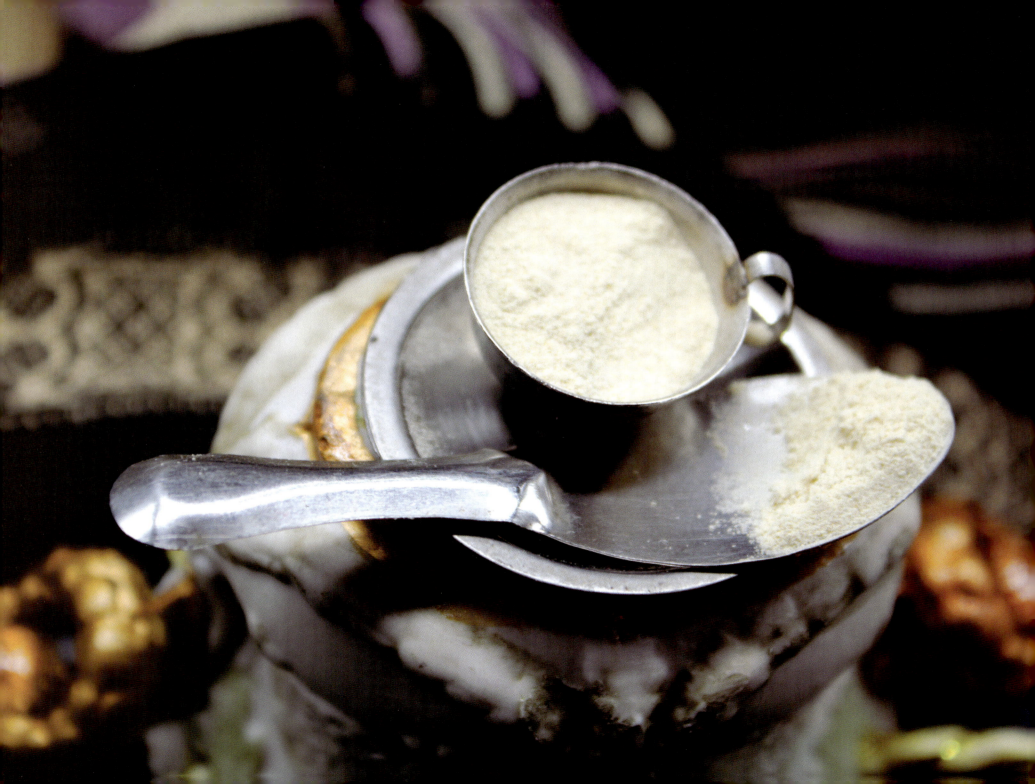

78. Āmḷānu Pāṇī (Natural Fat Burner Tea)

આમળાનું પાણી

To Boost metabolism, Promotes weight loss

- Place 1¼ cups of **WATER** in a pot on medium flame

- Add 1 teaspoon of **ORGANIC INDIAN GOOSEBERRY** (also known as **AMLA POWDER**). Optional: add 1 teaspoon of **ORGANIC TURMERIC POWDER**

- Mix well and when water comes to a boil, turn off the heat

- Pour into a mug and drink hot (not burning hot)

- Enjoy this Ayurvedic tea on an empty stomach first thing in the morning

- Repeat daily as needed

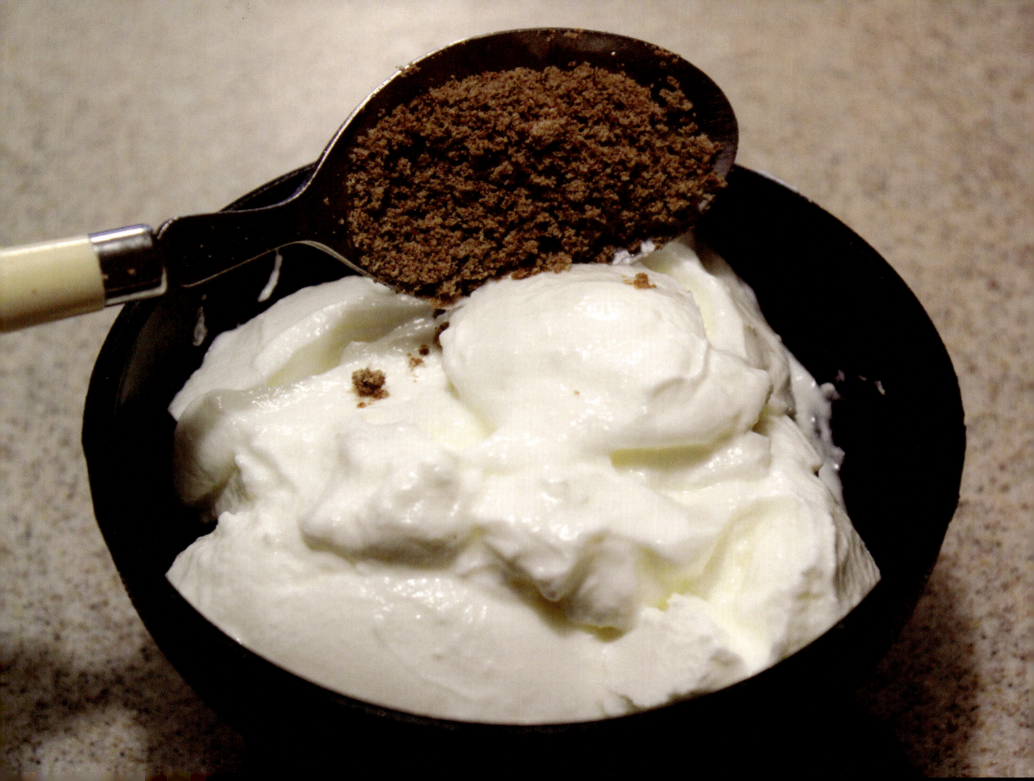

79. Aḷsī anē Dahī (Powerhouse Flaxseeds with Curd)
અળસી અને દહી

TO IMPROVE METABOLISM

- Grind 1 teaspoon of **FLAX SEEDS** to a powder

- Sprinkle this powder in a ½ cup of **YOGURT** of your choice

- Mix well

- Enjoy this during breakfast

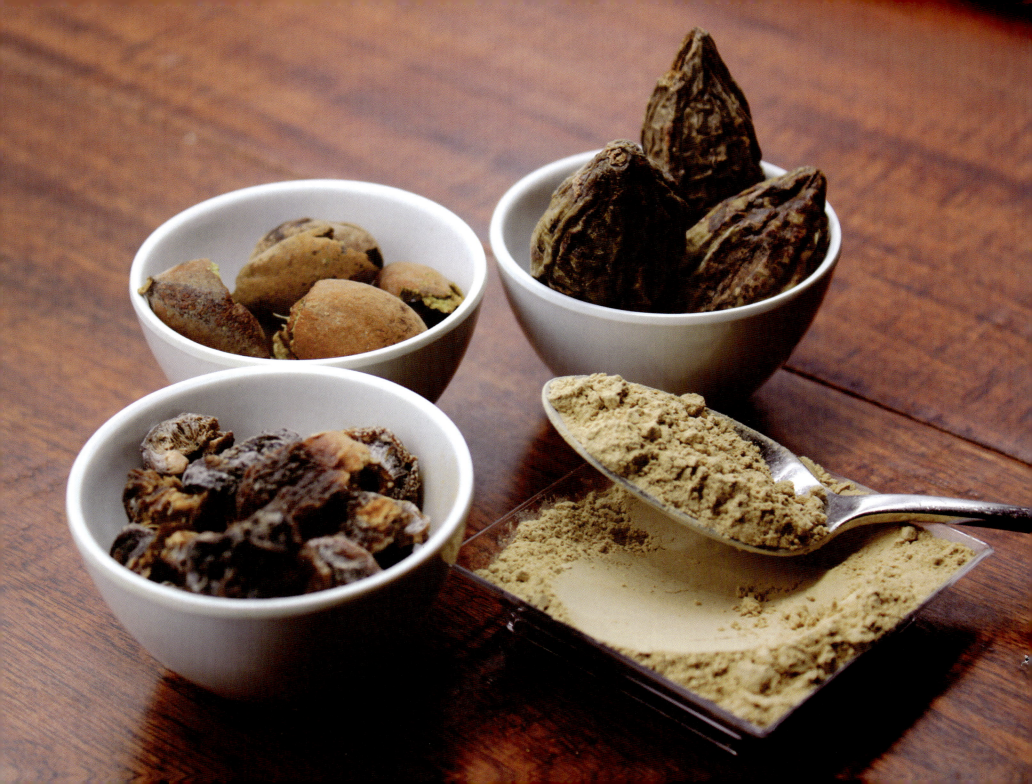

80. Trifaḷānu Pāṇī (Triphala Tea Infusion)

ત્રિફળાનું પાણી

To improve metabolism, weight loss

- Heat 1 cup of **WATER** in a pan

- Add ½ - 1 teaspoon of **ORGANIC TRIPHALA POWDER**

- Stir well and allow the powder to infuse in the hot water for 20 minutes

- Pour in a glass and drink on an empty stomach first thing in the morning

- Gulp any remaining powder that settled to the bottom of the glass

- Take this infusion <u>once a week with a lower dosage</u>

- Pay attention to your body and increase slowly to suggested dosage level

- Repeat daily and regulate dosage amount as your body feels comfortable

- Note: this tea infusion can be consumed on an empty stomach first thing in the morning (or about two hours after dinner and at least 30 minutes before going to bed)

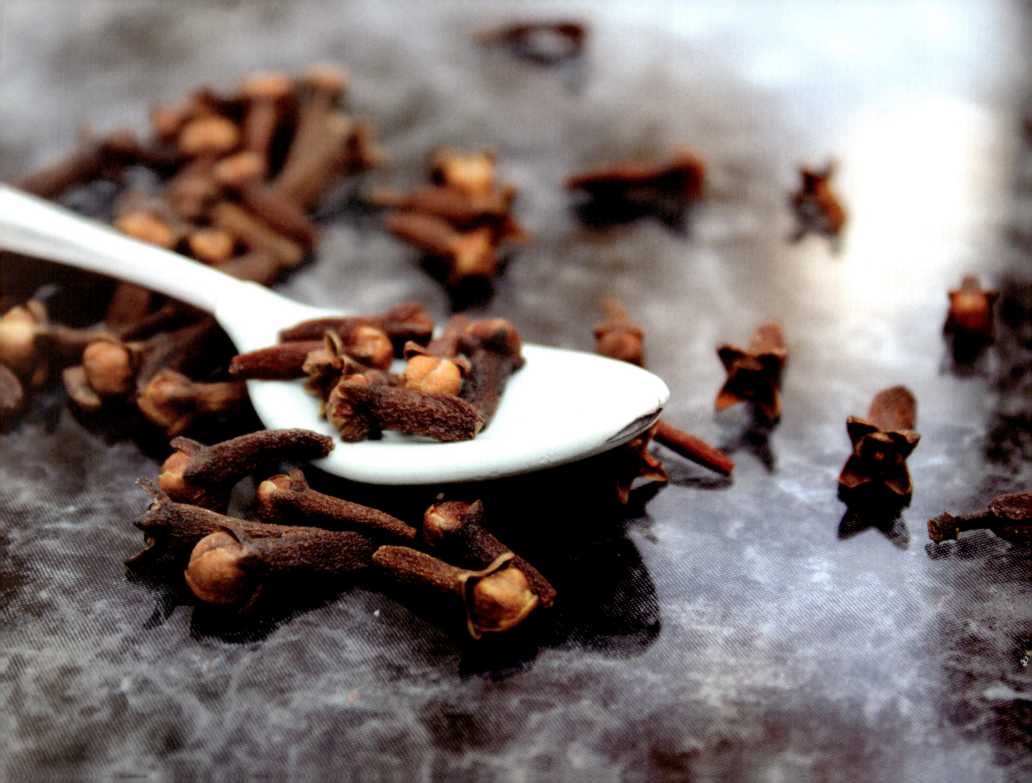

81. Lavīṅg Chāvavu (Relaxing Clove Gum)

લવીંગ ચાવવું

HELPS TO FIGHT MOTION SICKNESS

- Remove the bud (top section) of one **CLOVE**

- Suck on the clove stem for 30-60 minutes before you start on your journey

- Chew and swallow, or throw out the clove

- Repeat as needed during the trip

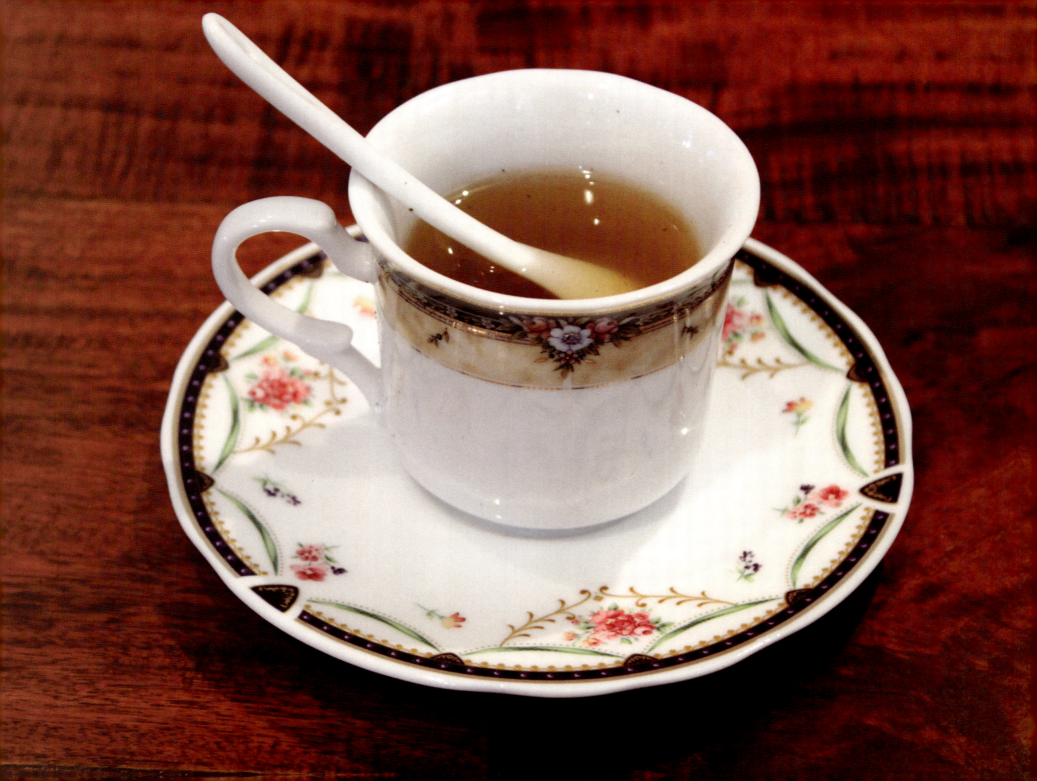

82. Madh anē Marī (Honey 'n Pepper Detox Tea)

મધ અને મરી

HELPS TO FIGHT DRY COUGH, DRAINS MUCUS

- Heat 8 ounces of **WATER** in a small pot on low flame
- Bring the water to a boil
- Grind 1 teaspoon of fresh **BLACK PEPPERCORN**
- Add 2 tablespoons of **ORGANIC HONEY** and powdered black peppercorn to the pot
- Mix these ingredients well and turn off the heat
- Let it <u>steep for 5 minutes</u>
- Strain into a mug using a metal sieve
- Enjoy this tea slowly while hot
- Repeat 2 times a day as needed

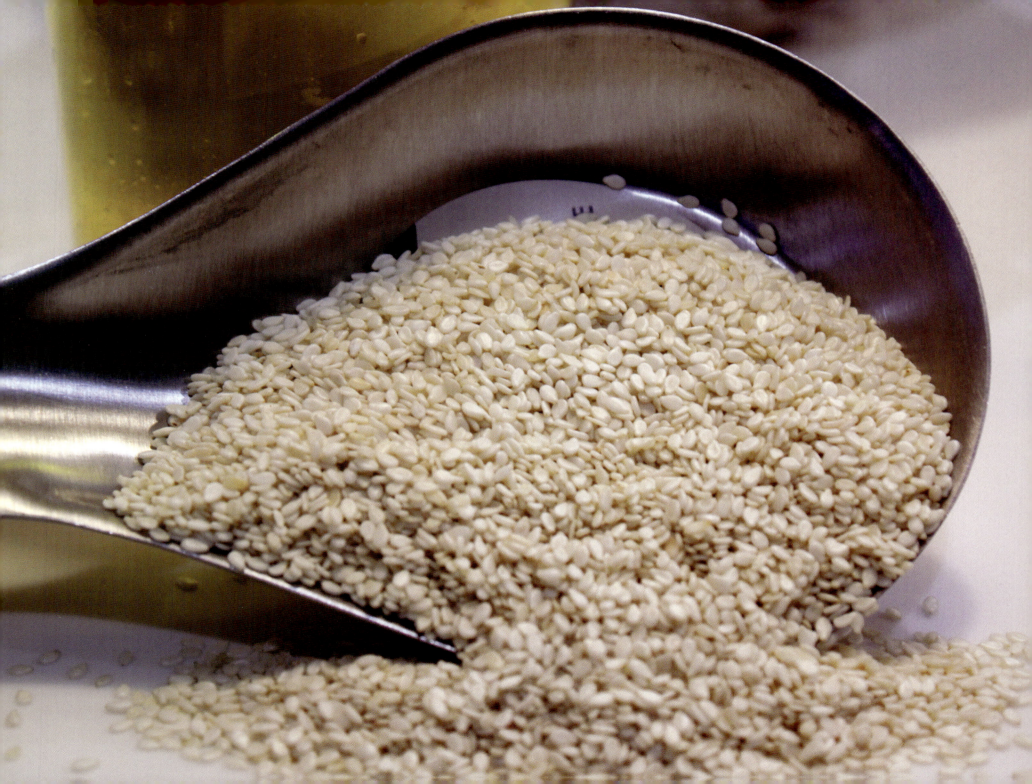

83. Tēl Māliśh (Sesame Oil Ayurvedic Massage)
તેલ માલિશ

RELIEF FROM MUSCLE SORENESS, JOINT PAIN, LEG SWELLING

- Wash your hands

- Lightly warm 2 tablespoons of **ORGANIC SESAME OIL** by holding it under a flame for 8-10 seconds, then let it cool

- Topically apply the oil on the skin to massage sore muscles, joints, tendons and swollen areas

- Using gentle pressure from your hands, <u>rub and massage oil for 5-10 minutes</u>

  - In circular motion over affected area (if problem is in a smaller area of the body)

  - In downward direction from top of affected area to bottom of affected area (if problem is a larger region of the body)

- Wash hands thoroughly afterward

- Repeat daily as needed

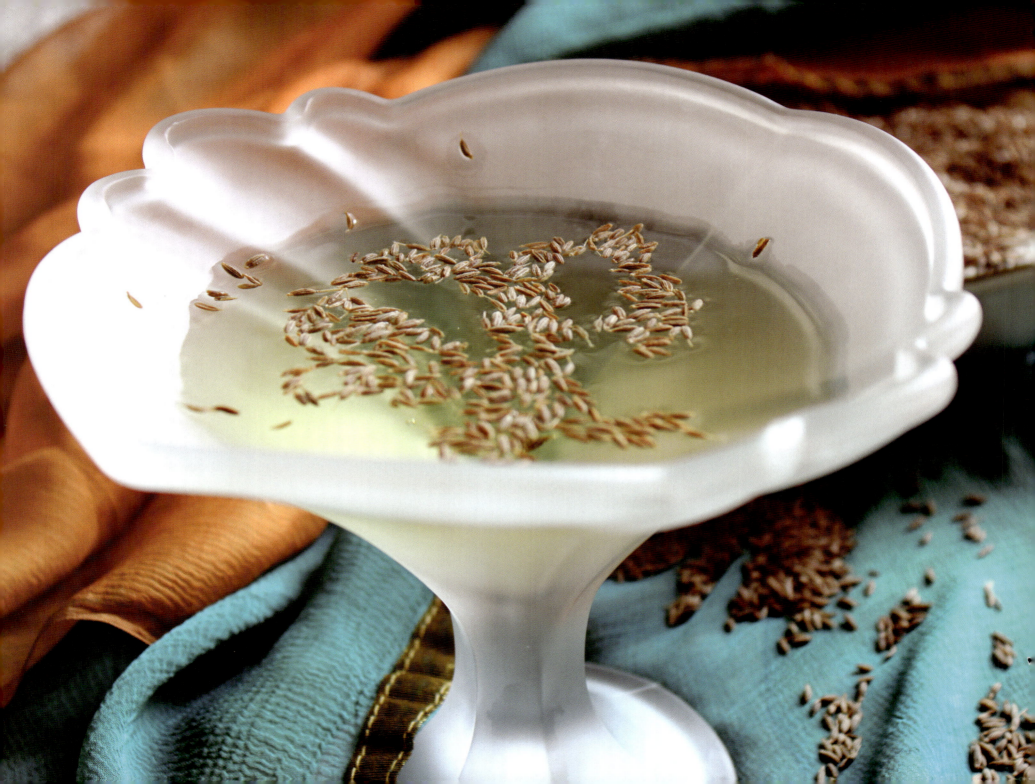

84. Jeerānu Pāṇī (Cumin Infused Tea)
જીરાનું પાણી

SOOTHES NAUSEA AND VOMITING

- Add 1 cup of **WATER** in a pot at medium flame

- Bring to a boil

- Add 1 teaspoon of **CUMIN SEEDS** and cover with a lid

- Immediately turn off the heat and let the cumin water steep for 5 minutes

- Mix well and pour into a mug

- Sip this piping hot drink slowly while hot and <u>chew the seeds</u>

- Repeat as needed and remember to stay hydrated

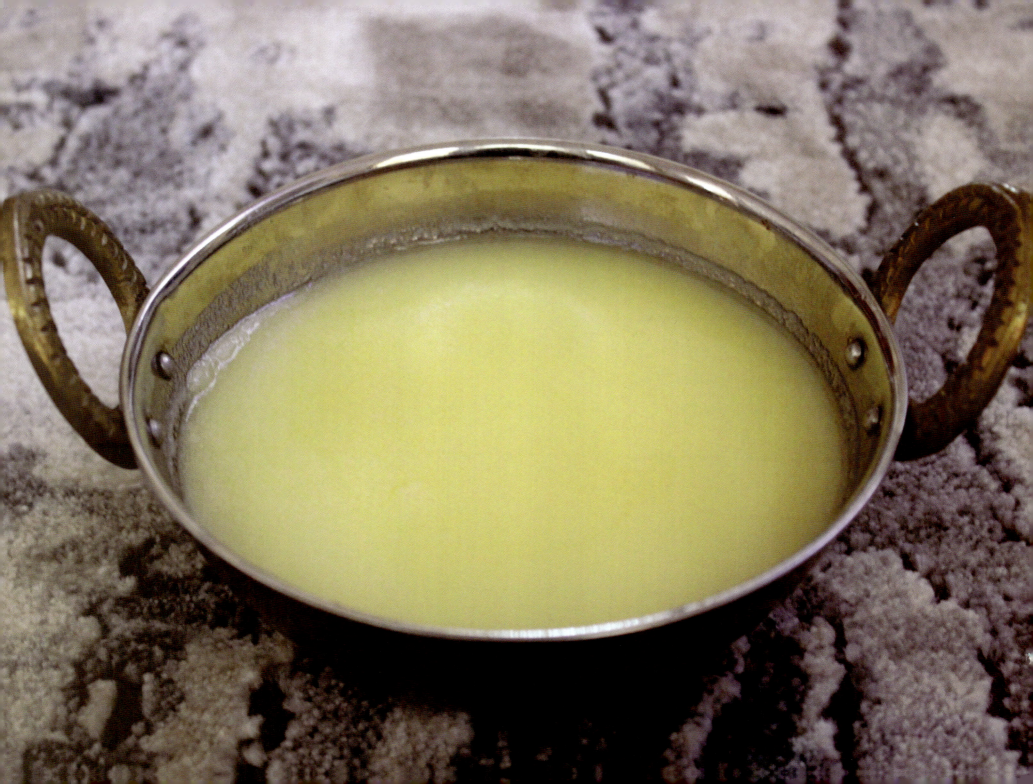

85. Ghee Nāak Mātē (Ghee Nose Ointment)

ધી નાક માટે

STOP THE NOSE BLEEDING

- Wash your hands

- Warm ¼ teaspoon of **GHEE** under a flame

- Let it cool

- Place a drop of cooled ghee in each nostril (via a dropper or a clean finger to gently insert into nostril)

- Repeat for <u>both nostrils in the morning and evening</u>

- Continue daily as needed

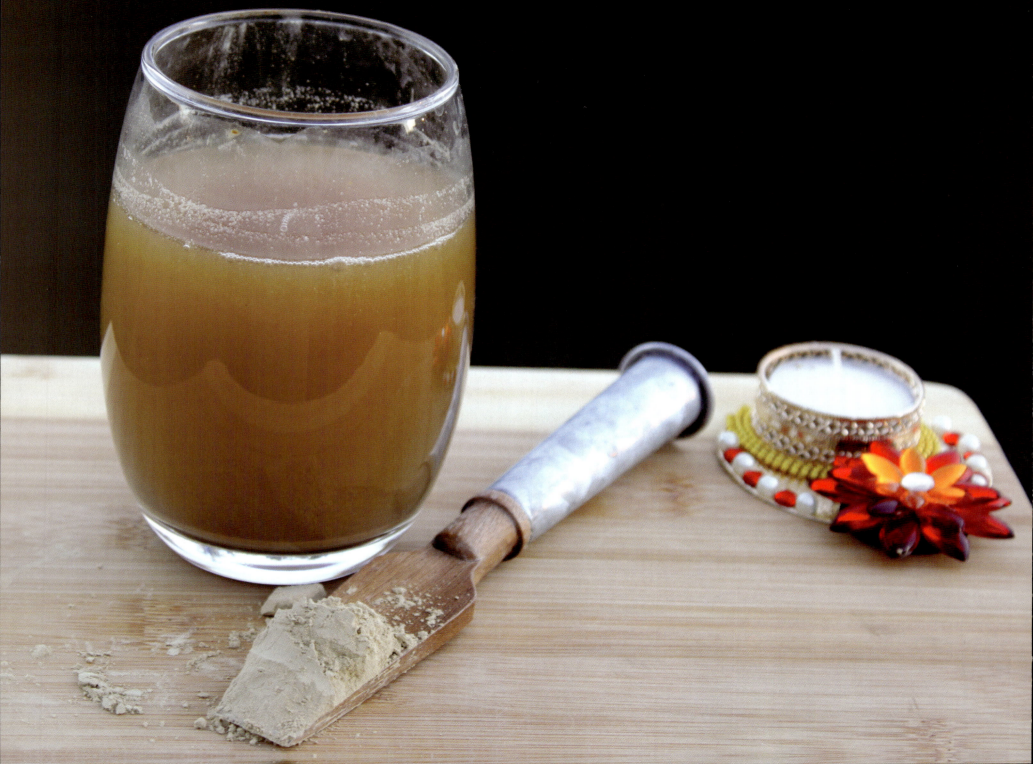

86. Trifaḷānā Kōglā (Triphala Mouth Wash)

ત્રિફળાના કોગળા

ORAL HEALTH, REDUCES PLAQUE, CAVITIES AND GUM INFLAMMATION

- Warm 1 cup of **WATER** in a pan on medium flame
- Mix ½ teaspoon of **ORGANIC TRIPHALA POWDER**
- Remove from heat after 1 minute
- When it cools, filter with a strainer into a cup
- Pour it into your mouth and <u>swish vigorously</u> for a full 30 seconds so that the triphala water comes in contact with all areas of your teeth, gums, under your tongue and across the roof of your moth
- Gargle for 30 seconds
- Spit out the triphala water into the sink
- Continue this process until all the water is empty
- Repeat this as part of your daily hygiene routine

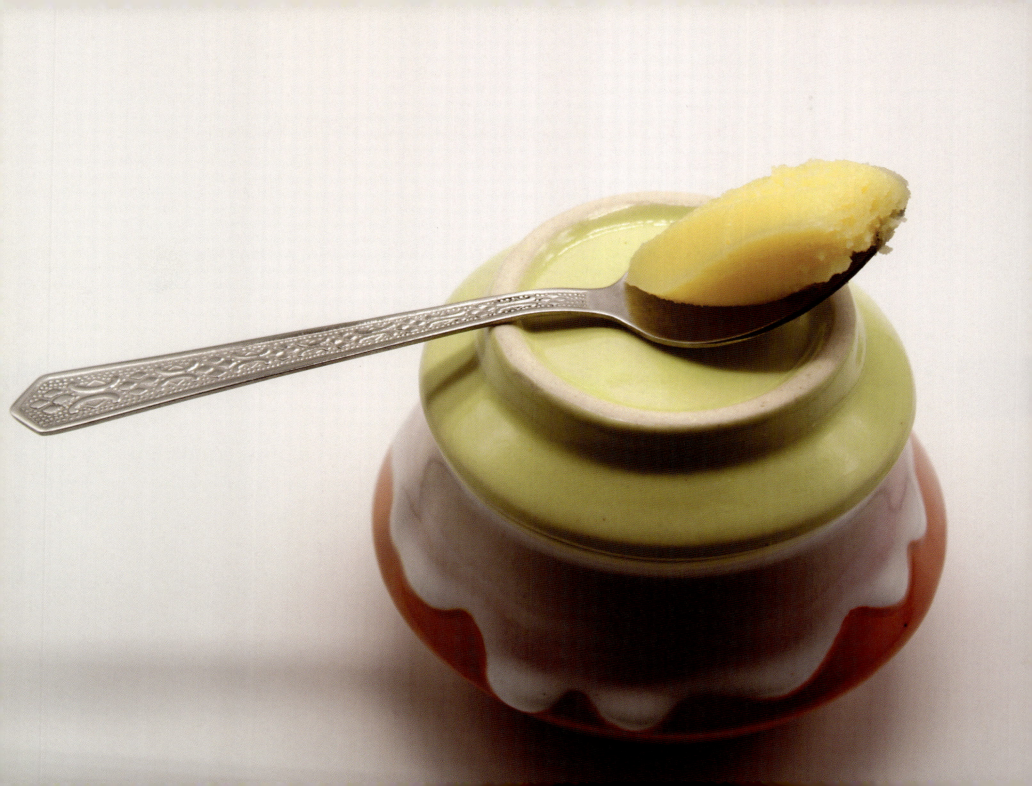

87. Ḍooṭī Upar Māliśh (Therapeutic Belly Button Massage)

ડ્રૂટી ઉપર માલિશ

IMPROVES POOR VISION, RELIEVES DRY EYES , SOFTENS SKIN, KEEPS HAIR SILKY

- Wash your hands

- Warm 1 tablespoon **PURE ORGANIC GHEE** on low flame

- When it is lukewarm (safe to touch), pour the ghee into a dropper

- Lie down on a flat surface. Use the dropper to slowly place 3 drops of warm ghee in the belly button (naval pit) and spread it 1 and half inches around the naval area with your fingers

- Gently massage the naval area in a clockwise direction for 3-5 minutes and with a counter-clockwise motion for another 3-5 minutes

- Enjoy this splendid, magical massage during bedtime on nightly basis

- Note: do not perform this warm ghee belly bath on a full stomach and keep a gap of at least 2 hours after eating

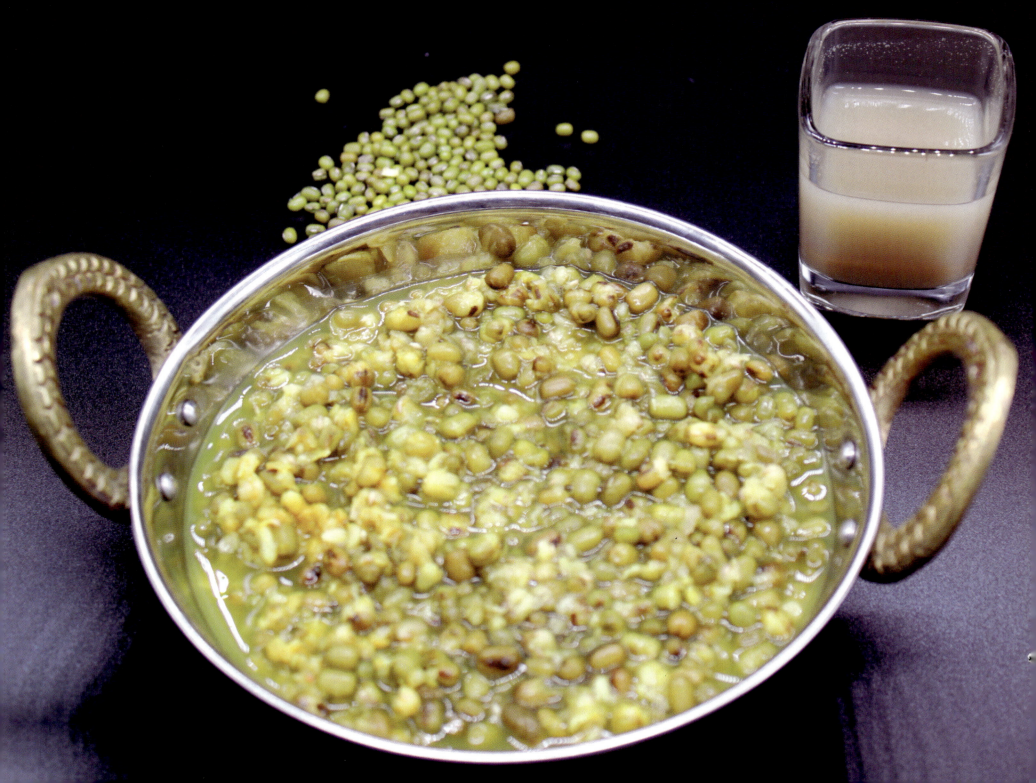

88. Moongnu Pāṇī (Moong Detox Soup)
મગનું પાણી

FOR PROTEIN BOOST, AFTER COMPLETION OF A FAST

- Thoroughly wash and rinse ½ cup of **MOONG BEANS** and let soak for 30 minutes

- Rinse water and add soaked moong beans to pressure cooker with 1½ cups **WATER**

- Add ½ teaspoon **SALT** and ½ teaspoon **GROUND ORGANIC TURMERIC POWDER**

- Close the lid and cook the moong beans on medium flame for 3 whistles (optional: this can be cooked in a pot - double water ratio to 3 cups and let the beans cook for 30 minutes til soft to touch)

- Turn off stove, lightly mash beans and strain liquid portion (moong water) in a cup

- Set aside the cooked moong beans in a bowl

- Melt 1 teaspoon of **GHEE**, add to the cup of moong water and mix well

- Slowly drink this detox soup then enjoy the bowl of cooked moong beans while hot

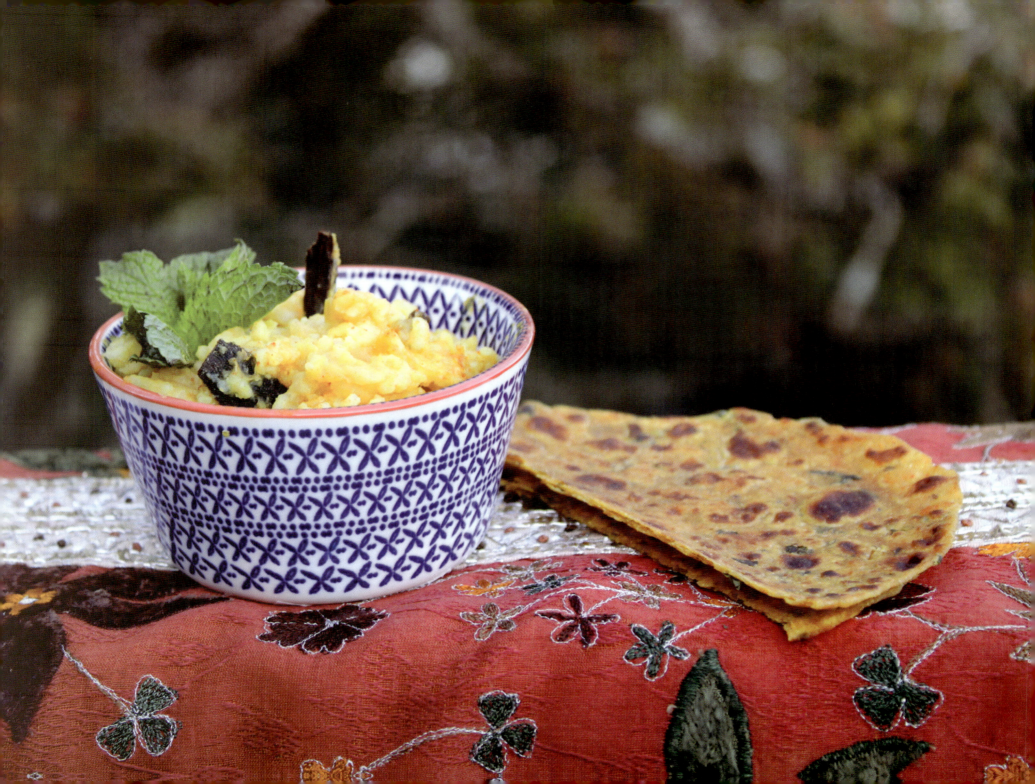

89. Tuvēr Dāḷnī Khīchaḍī (Rice and Lentil Super Food)

તુવેર દાળની ખીચડી

FOR PROTEIN BOOST AND GENERAL HEALTH

- Wash and soak ½ cup **RICE** and ½ cup **SPLIT PIGEON PEAS DAL/LENTIL**

- In a small pressure cooker heat **GHEE** on low flame

- Add 1 **CINNAMON STICK**, 2 **CLOVES** and pinch of **ASAFOETIDA** and sauté these ingredients

- Add soaked dal/lentil, rice ½ teaspoon **RED CHILI POWDER**, ¼ teaspoon **GROUND ORGANIC TURMERIC POWDER** and **SALT** to taste

- Add 2 cups of **WATER**, mix it well and bring to a rolling boil on high heat

- Close lid on pressure cooker, reduce heat to medium and pressure cook for 3 whistles

- Remove from the heat and <u>allow the pressure to naturally release</u> before opening the lid

- Mix gently and pour a teaspoon of ghee on top to enhance the flavors

- Serve this powered comfort food in a plate or bowl.

- Enjoy while hot with **YOGURT** of your choice or roasted **PAPADUM**

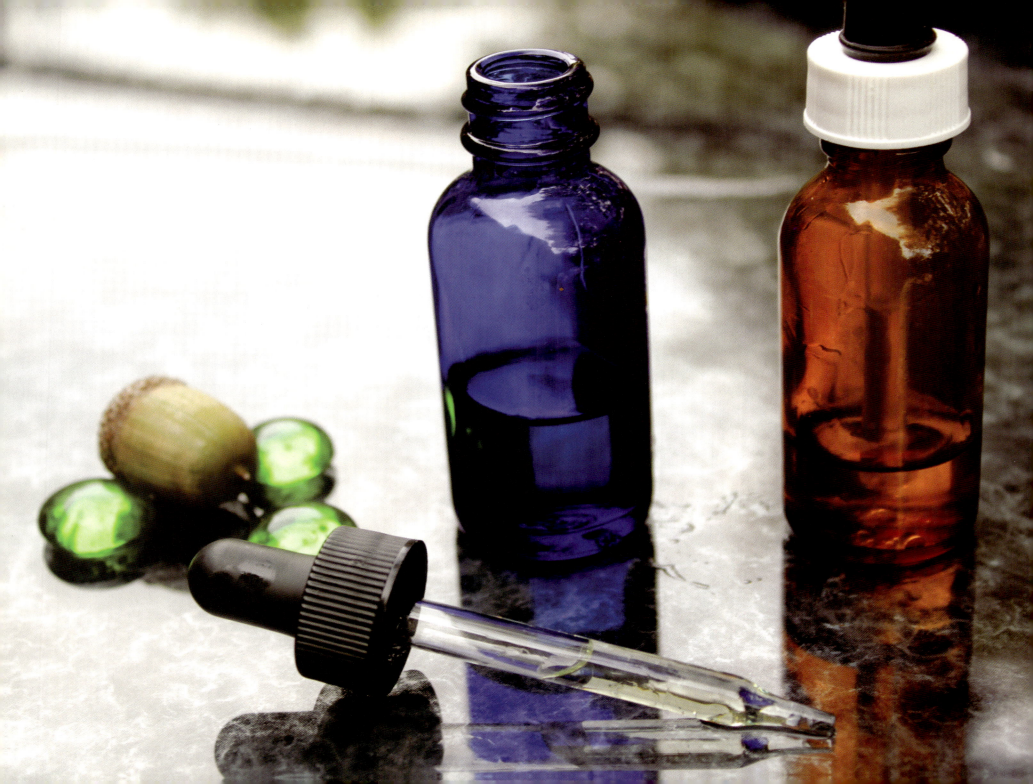

90. Deevēl Māliśh (Castor Oil Lotion)

દીવેલ માલિશ

FOR RELIEF FROM RASH ON SKIN OR DIAPER RASH

- Wash your hands

- Pour a couple drops of **CASTOR OIL** on your fingers

- Apply the oil to <u>coat the affected area</u>

- Rub the oil gently with your fingers

- Repeat as needed

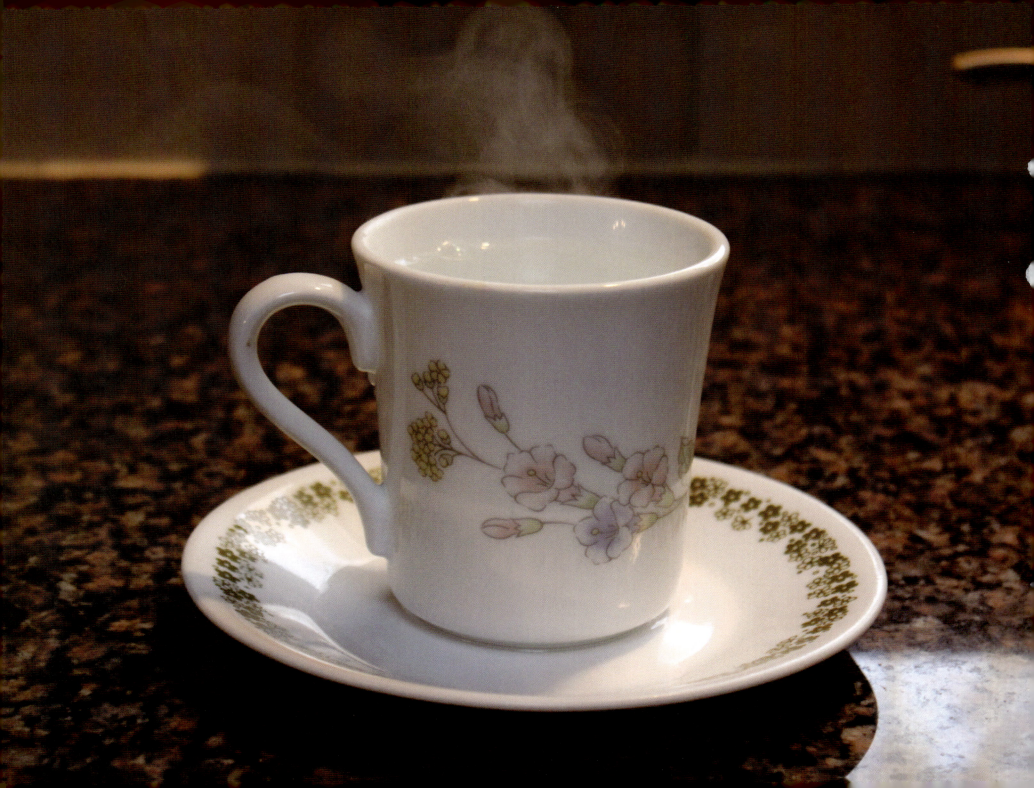

91. Navśhēku Pāṇī (Lukewarm Water Routine)
નવશેકુ પાણી

FOR REGULAR BOWEL MOVEMENT

- Drink 2-3 glasses of **LUKEWARM WATER** on an empty stomach first thing in the morning

- After drinking water, <u>wait 45 minutes</u> before eating any food

- Repeat daily

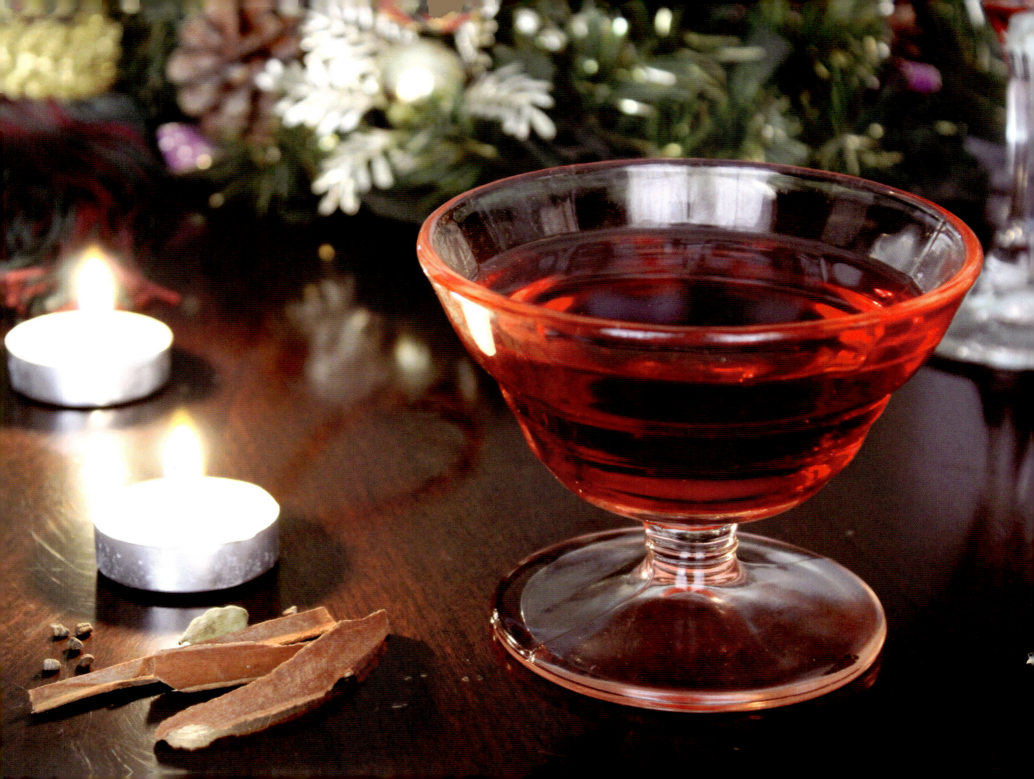

92. Sāakarnu Pāṇī (Refreshing Sweet Water)

સાકરનું પાણી

FOR REJUVENATION AFTER WATER FAST, RELIEF FROM COUGH WITH PHLEGM, CLEARS THROAT

- Add 1 cups of **WATER** in a pan to medium heat
- Let it come to a boil
- Remove pan from the heat and turn off the stove
- Crush 2 **ROCK SUGARS** using a mortal & pestle to a fine pulverized powder to fill 1 tablespoon
- Add powdered rock sugar to the pan and stir until the sugar fully dissolves
- Add 1 **CLOVE**, 1 small **CINNAMON STICK** and a pinch of **CARDAMOM POWDER**
- Close the lid and <u>let it cool for 1 hour</u>
- Sieve the water
- Pour in a glass and enjoy this rejuvenating, spiced rock sugar drink

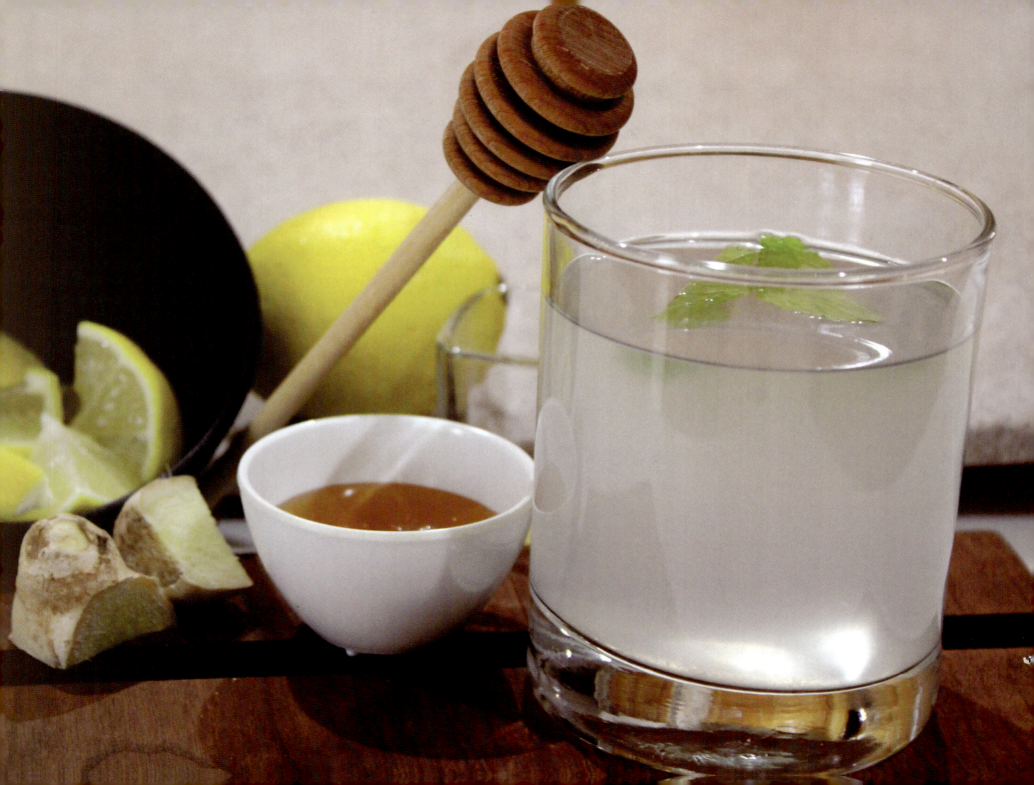

93. Madh anē Āadu (Honey Ginger Solution)
મધ અને આદુ

TREAT RUNNY NOSE, LOOSEN PHLEGM, DECONGESTANT

- Wash your hands

- Peel 1 inch of fresh **GINGER** and grate onto a plate

- Squeeze the grated ginger using your finger to extract juice into a small bowl

- Add 1 teaspoon of **HONEY** into the juice of ginger

- Mix well and take a spoonful in your mouth

- Swallow very slowly

- Avoid drinking water for 30 minutes after taking this solution

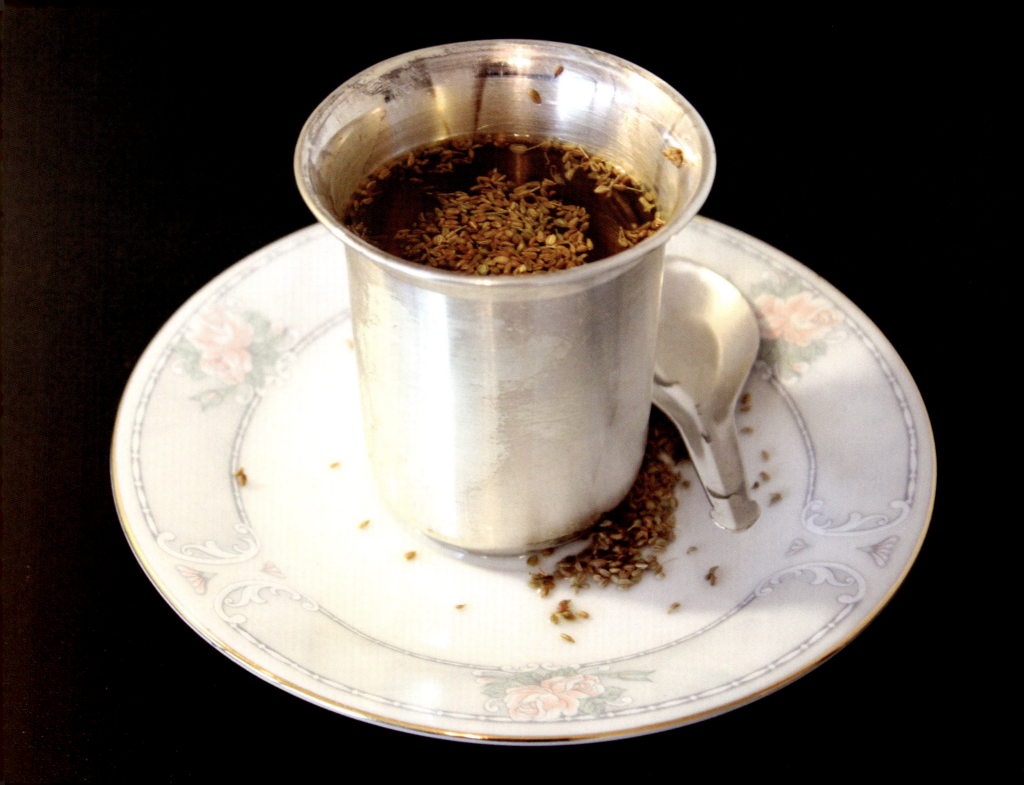

94. Ajmānu Pāṇī (Ajwain Water)

અજમાનું પાણી

FOR COUGH, COLD, SINUS, SORE THROAT

- Add 1 cup of **WATER** in a small pot
- Add 1 teaspoon of **AJWAIN SEEDS**
- Add ¼ teaspoon of **ORGANIC JAGGERY**
- Bring to a boil
- Turn off the stove and sprinkle a <u>pinch</u> of **SALT**
- Stir and enjoy while hot

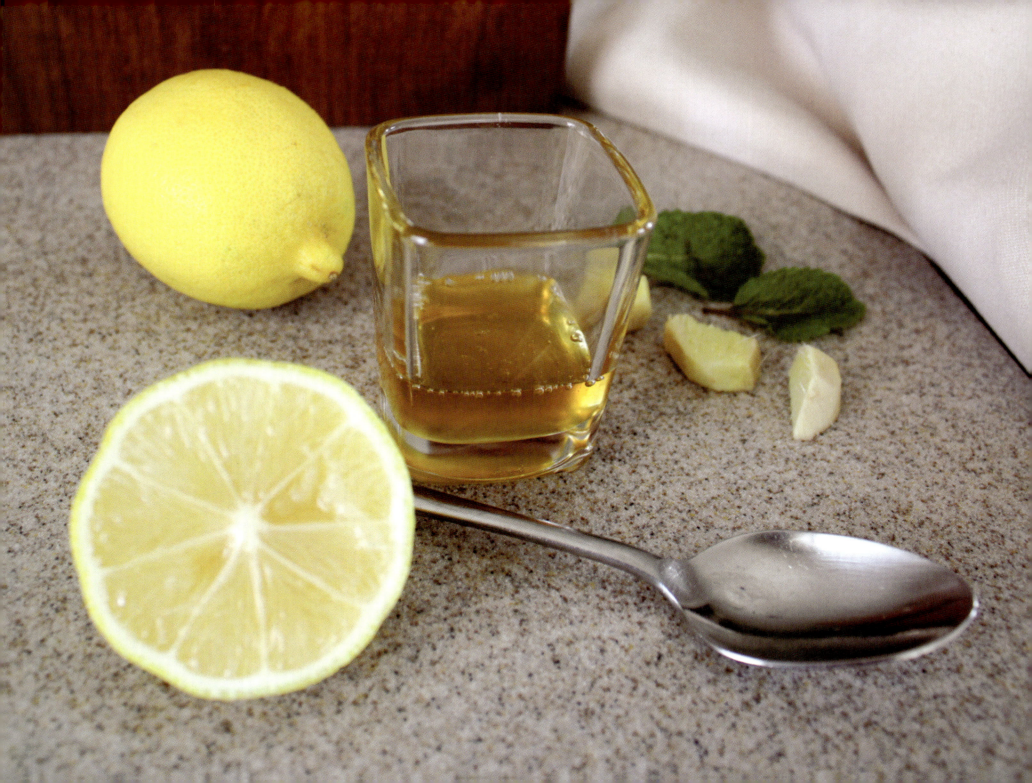

95. Āadu Līmbunō Rus (Soothing Lemon Ginger Tea)

આદુ લીંબુનો રસ

TO SOOTHE THROAT DURING COUGH, COLD, SINUS OR CONGESTION

- Peel 1 inch of fresh **GINGER** and cut into slices

- Put 1½ cups of **WATER** and sliced ginger to a small pot

- Cut fresh **LEMON** and squeeze 1 teaspoon of juice

- Add 1 teaspoon of **HONEY**

- Mix all the ingredients and bring to a boil

- Stir and strain the water

- Enjoy this drink while hot

- Repeat 3 times a day as needed for relief

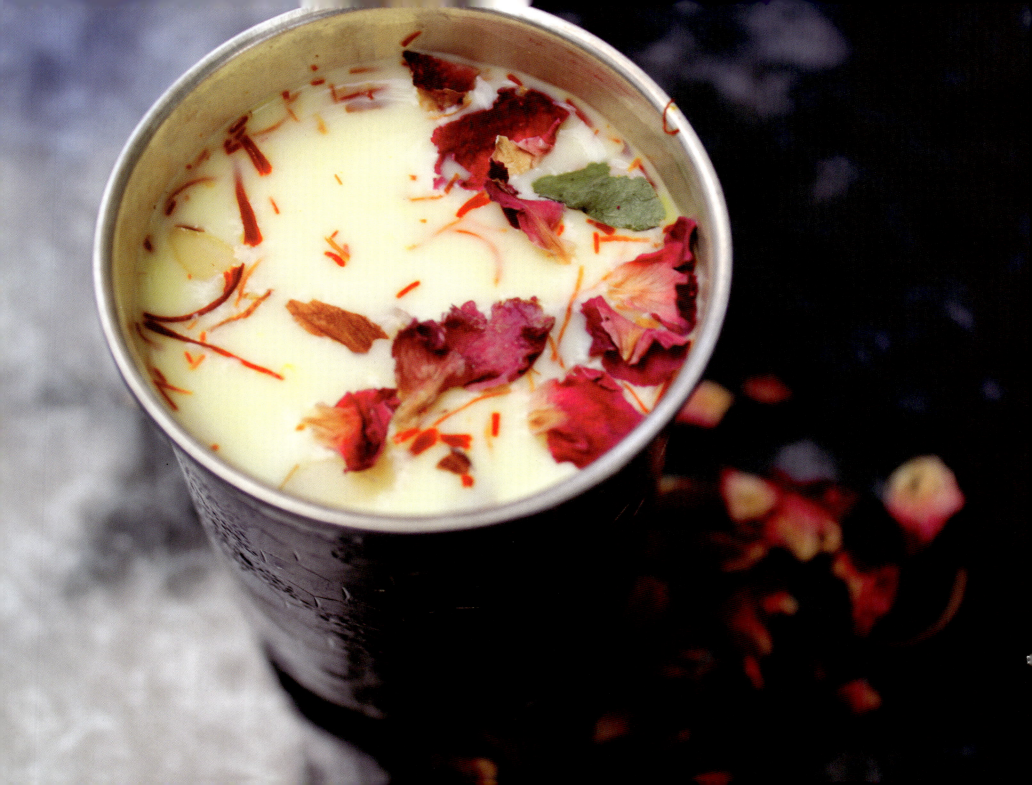

96. Kēsar Pīstānu Doodh (Aromatic Saffron Latte)

કેસર પીસ્તાનું દૂધ

RELAXES SORE MUSCLES

- Cut 3 **ORGANIC WHOLE ALMONDS** and 2 **ORGANIC PISTACHIOS** into fine slivers, and set aside

- Pour 1 cup **MILK** of your choice to a small pot and heat over low heat

- Add 1½ teaspoons of **SUGAR** of your preference

- Add a pinch of **CARDAMOM POWDER**

- Take 4 small threads of **SAFFRON** and gently crush to a powder state using your fingers

- Add saffron, slivered almonds and slivered pistachios

- Stir until flavors blend

- Bring to a boil and let it <u>simmer for 1 minute</u>

- Pour into a mug

- Enjoy this soothing latte piping hot or as a chilled nourishing refresher

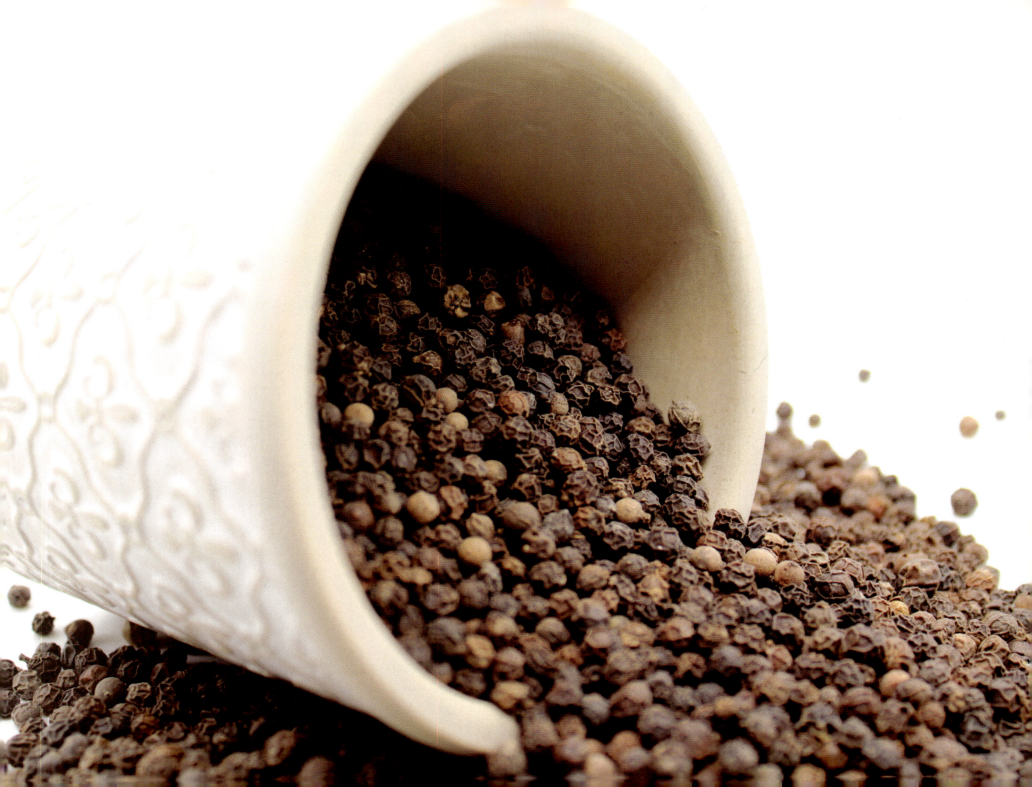

97. Kālā Marī (Peppery Toffee Lozenge)

કાળા મરી

TO ALLEVIATE SORE THROAT

- Grind ¼ teaspoon of fresh **BLACK PEPPERCORN** into a small bowl
- Add 1 teaspoon of **ORGANIC HONEY** and mix well
- Consume this mixture in your mouth and swallow very slowly
- Avoid drinking water for 30 minutes after taking this solution

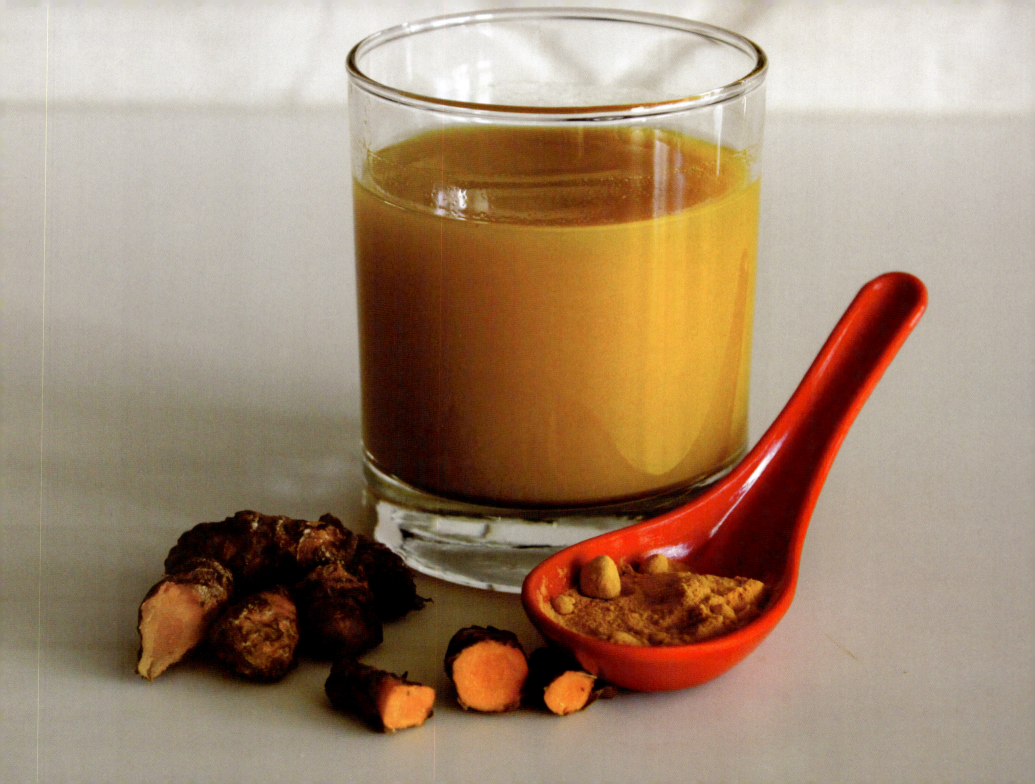

98. Haḷdarnu Pāṇī (Golden Turmeric Water)

હળદરનું પાણી

EXCELLENT FOR COUGH, COLD, SINUS, SORE THROAT

- Heat 1 teaspoon of **PURE ORGANIC GHEE** in a small pot on medium flame
- Sauté ½ teaspoon **GROUND ORGANIC TURMERIC POWDER**
- Immediately add 1½ cups of **WATER**
- Stir <u>continuously</u> and bring to a boil
- Add ¼ teaspoon of **SALT**
- Pour into a mug and stir
- Enjoy this soothing drink while hot
- Repeat daily as needed

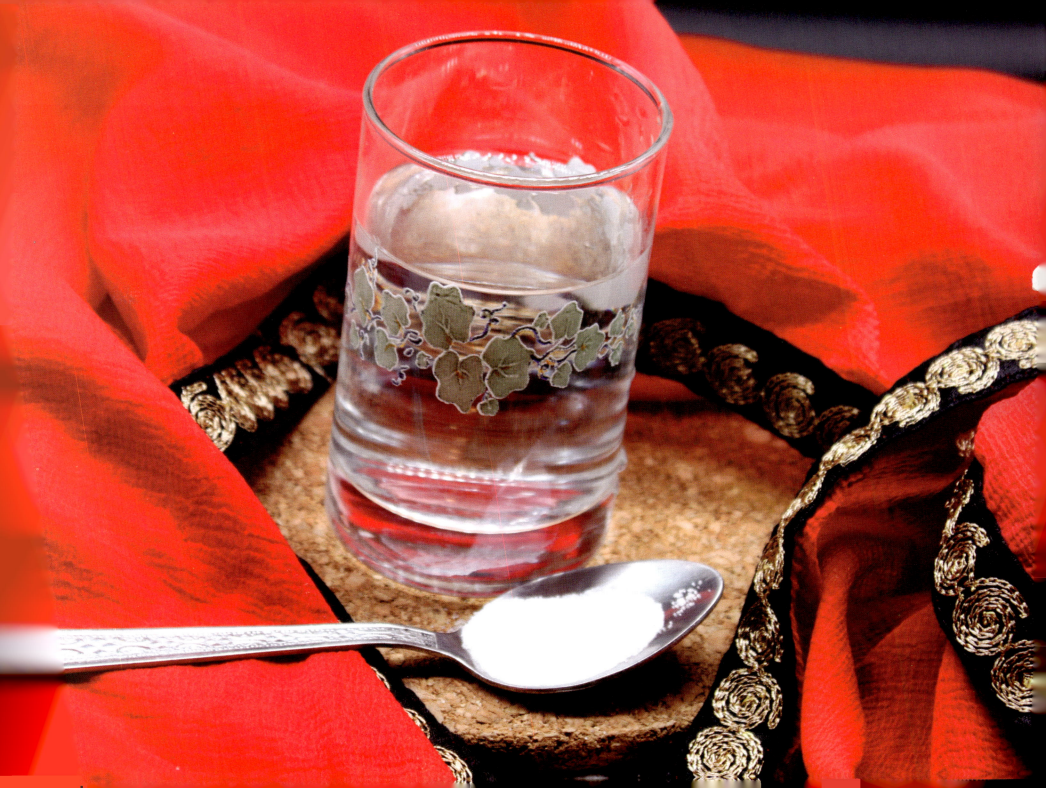

99. Mīṭhānā Pāṇīna Kōgla (Salt Water Gargle)
મીઠાના પાણીના કોગળા

BENEFICIAL FOR SORE THROAT, REDUCES THROAT IRRITATION

- Boil 8 ounces of **WATER** on a pot at medium flame

- Stir 1 teaspoon of **SALT** and mix thoroughly until the salt has dissolved

- When water is warm to touch, take a large sip of this solution in your mouth

- Tilt your head back

- Gargle for 20-30 seconds

- Swish the water in your mouth

- Spit out the water in sink

- Continue this process until all the water is finished

- Repeat salt water gargle every 2-3 hours as needed

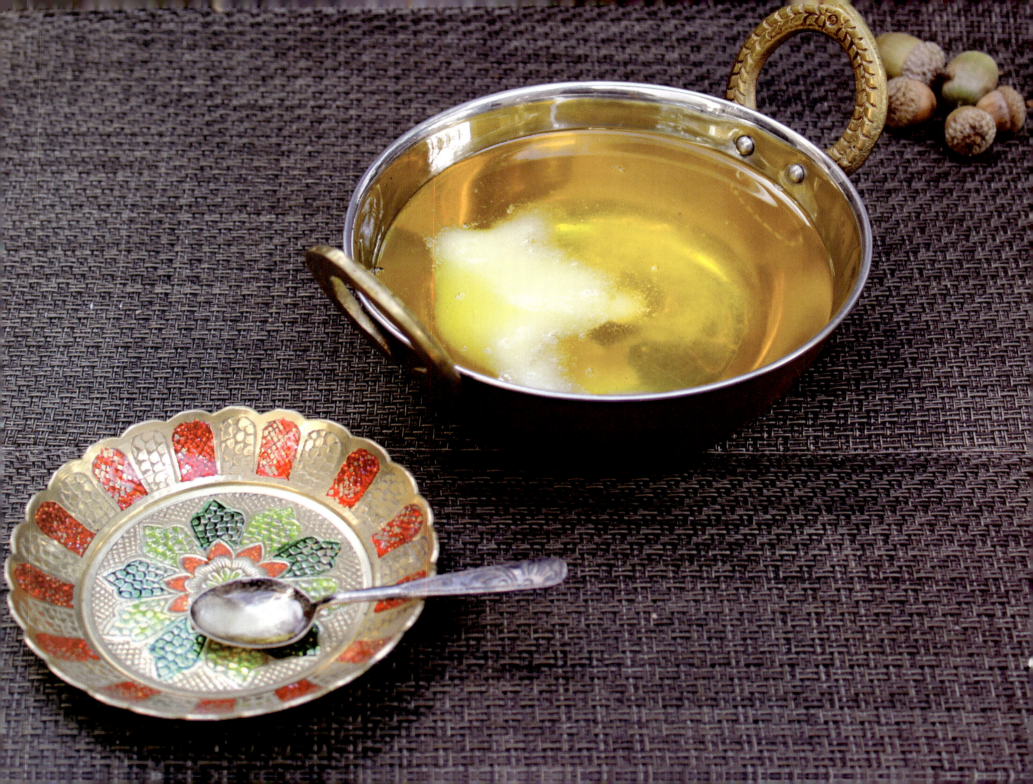

100. Vāaḷma Ghee Lagāvō (Ghee Hair Mask)

વાળમાં ઘી લગાવો

REDUCE SPLIT ENDS ON DRY HAIR

- Heat 4 tablespoons of **PURE ORGANIC GHEE** until it melts in a small pot on low heat

- Let it cool down until it is warm and safe to touch

- Massage the ghee to the bottom of hair locks (split ends)

- <u>After 1 hour</u> take a shower

- Wash your hair with a mild shampoo

- Rinse with water

- Repeat as needed

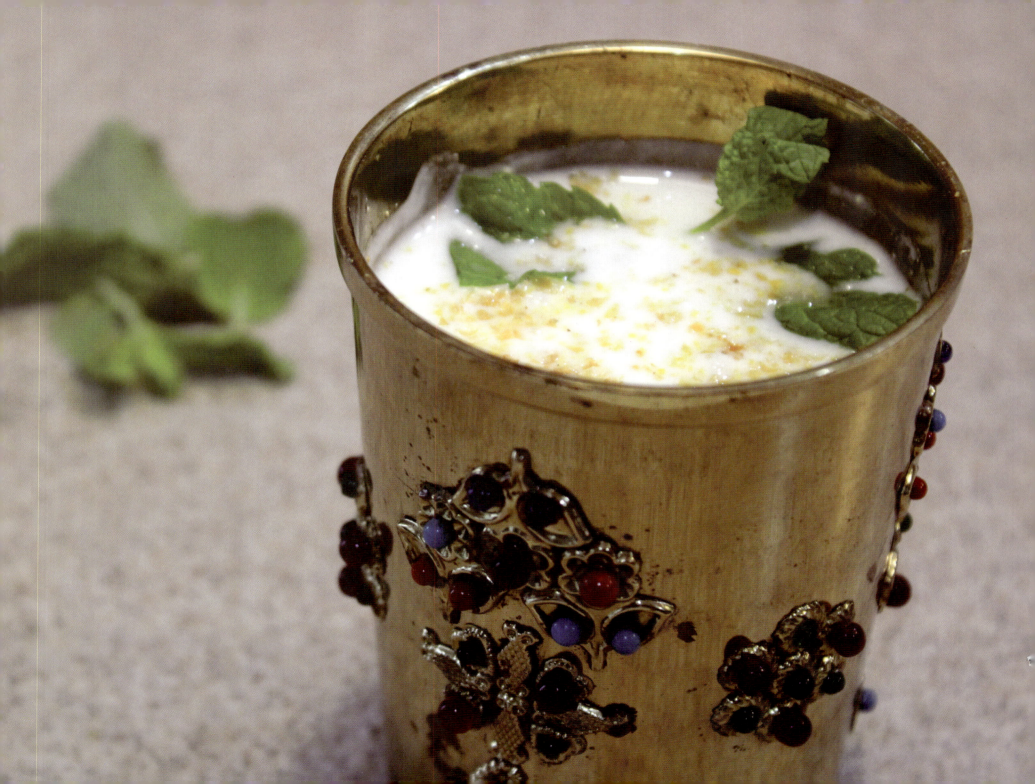

101. Mēthīnī Chhāś (Fenugreek Spiced Buttermilk)

મેથીની છાશ

TO REDUCE STOMACH ACHE

- Heat a non-stick pan on medium heat

- Sauté ½ teaspoon of **FENUGREEK SEEDS** for 2-3 minutes until color deepens into a dark brown color

- Use mortal and pestle (or grinder) to lightly crush the seeds to promote the release of flavor and aroma

- Blend crushed fenugreek seeds into an 8 ounce glass of **BUTTERMILK** (see Remedy 75 for buttermilk recipe)

- Stir and enjoy this savory spiced drink

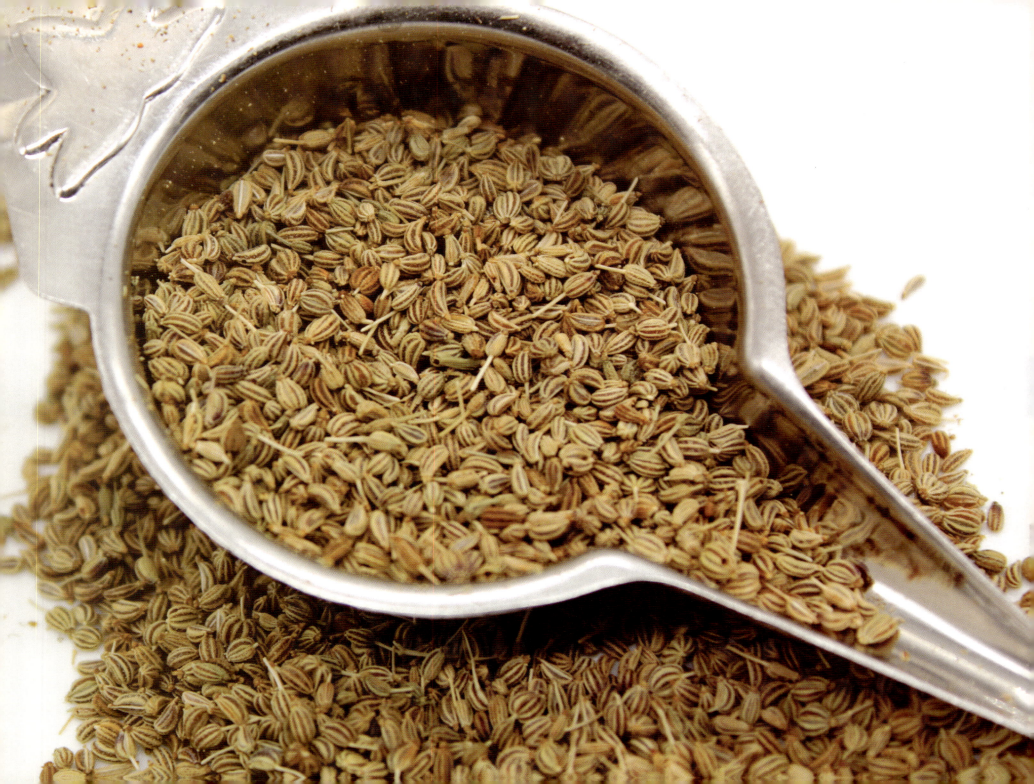

102. Ajmānī Fākī (Ajwain Syrup)

અજમાની ફાકી

IMMEDIATE RELIEF FROM STOMACH ACHE AND GAS

- Put ½ teaspoon of **AJWAIN SEEDS** and a pinch of **SALT** in mouth

- <u>Swallow</u> this mixture with ½ - 1 glass of **WATER**

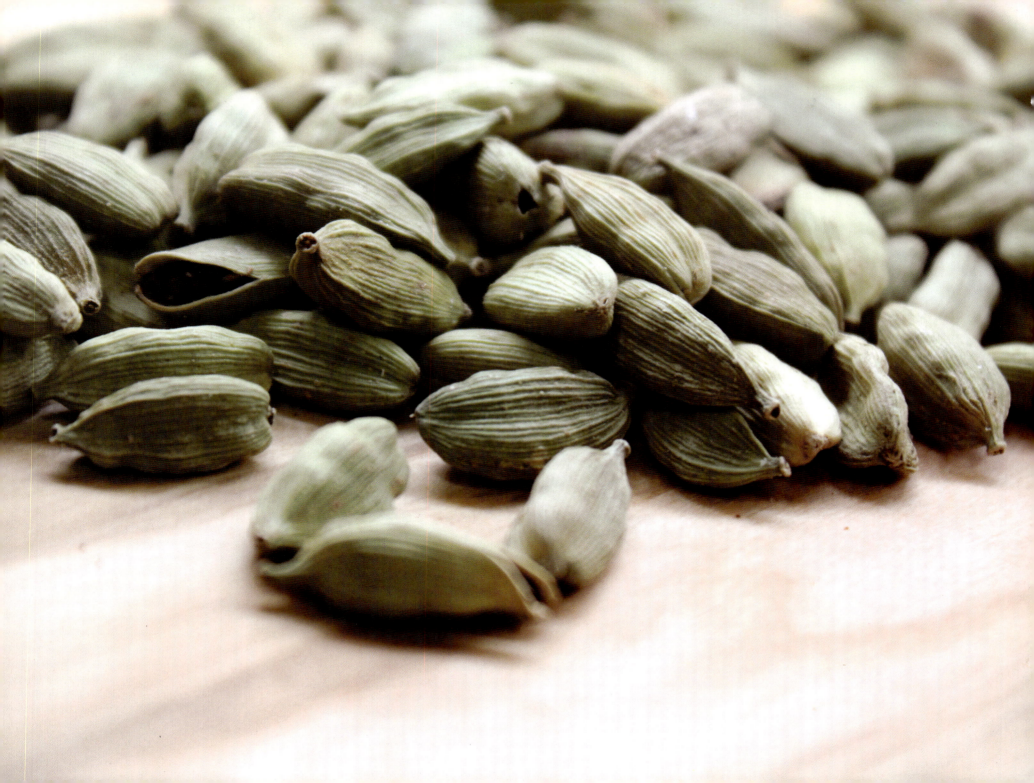

103. Elāichī Ghee (Cardamom Peepramul Syrup)

ઈલાયચી ઘી

RELIEVES STOMACH PAINS

- Grind seeds from one **CARDAMOM POD** until pulverized into fine powder and transfer to small bowl

- Add ¼ teaspoon of **PEEPRAMUL POWDER**

- Mix these spices well with ¼ teaspoon of **PURE ORGANIC GHEE**

- Take this mixture in your mouth

- Repeat as needed for relief

- <u>Avoid drinking water</u> for 30 minutes afterward

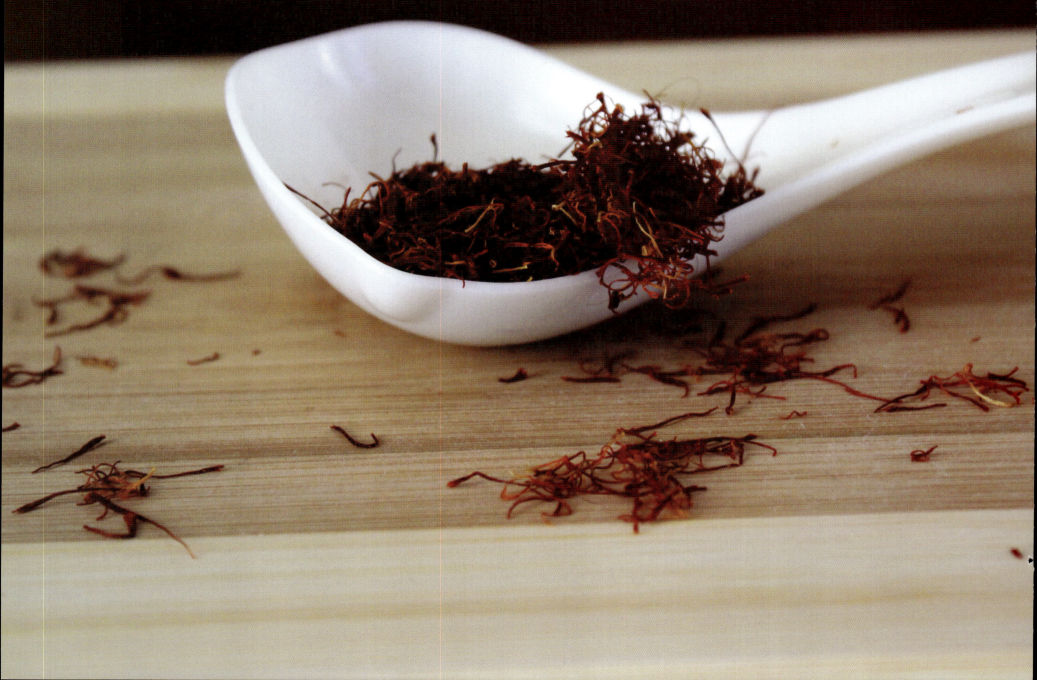

104. Kēsar (Anti-Inflammatory Saffron Healing Paste)

કેસર

HEALS EYE STYE

- Wash your hands

- Take 3 threads of **SAFFRON** and crush to powder form

- Add few drops of **WATER** and mix til it becomes thick paste

- Gently apply to affected area (<u>above or under eyelid</u>) with your finger. Avoid getting saffron paste inside the eye as it can cause irritation

- Let it dry for 15 minutes

- Carefully rinse out the paste

- Repeat this 2-3 times a day until you are healed

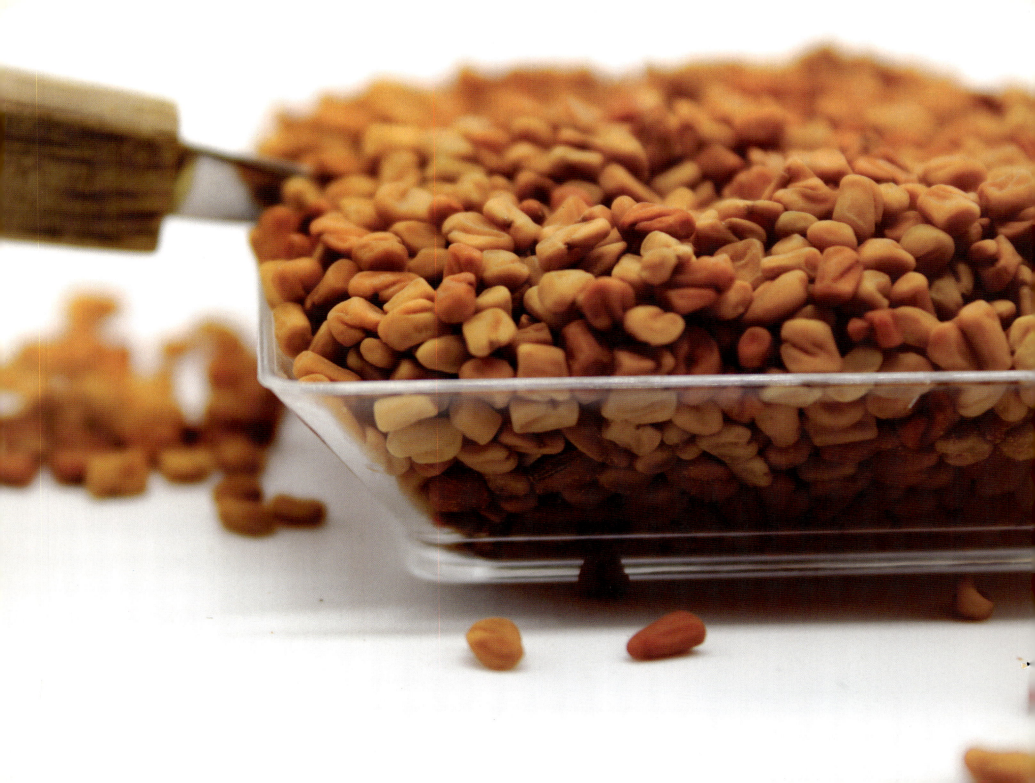

105. Mēthinā Dāṇā (Weight Loss Fenugreek Drink)

મેથીના દાણા

FOR WEIGHT LOSS

- Soak 1 tablespoon of **FENUGREEK SEEDS** into an 8 ounce glass of **WATER** overnight

- In the morning strain and filter the water in a bowl

- Chew the <u>soaked seeds</u> slowly first thing in the morning on an empty stomach

- Now drink the filtered water

- Repeat daily for at least 6 months

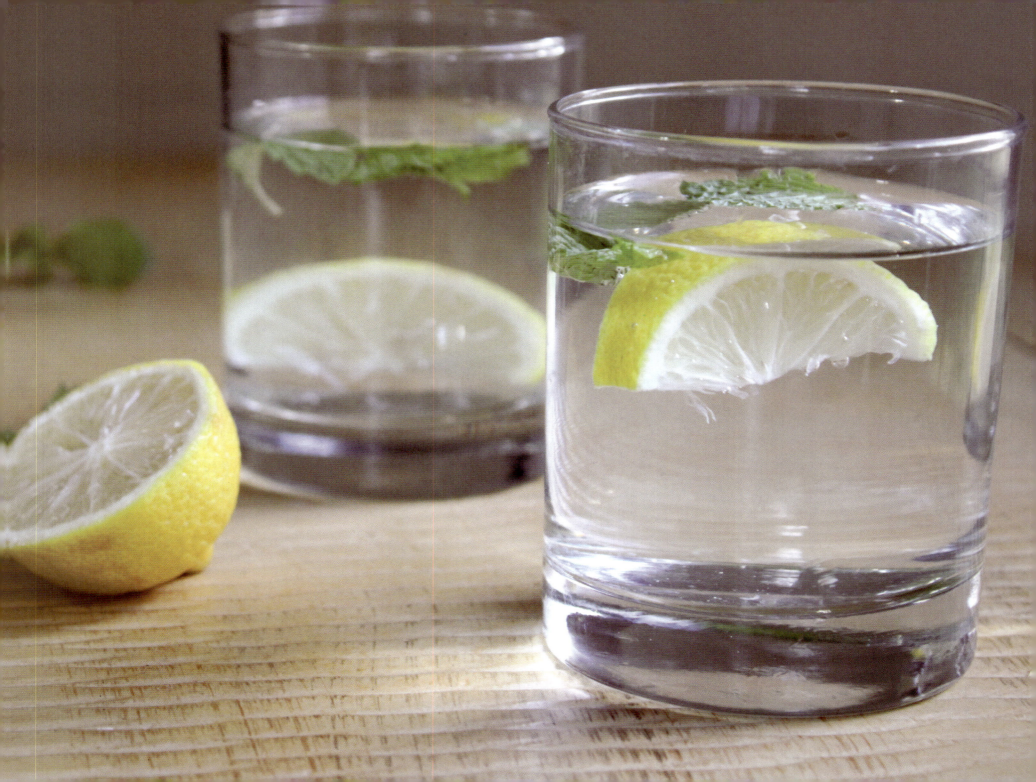

106. Līmbu anē Fudīnānu Pāṇī (Lemon-Infused Refresher)

લીંબુ અને ફુદીનાનું પાણી

LOWERS HEART DISEASE, PROMOTES WEIGHT LOSS, IMMUNITY BOOST

- Cut 3 thin slices of **LEMON**

- Pour room temperature **WATER** to a container and add the lemon slices (optional: add 1-2 sprigs of washed fresh **MINT LEAVES**)

- Mix and shake

- Drink this water <u>throughout</u> the day

- Repeat daily

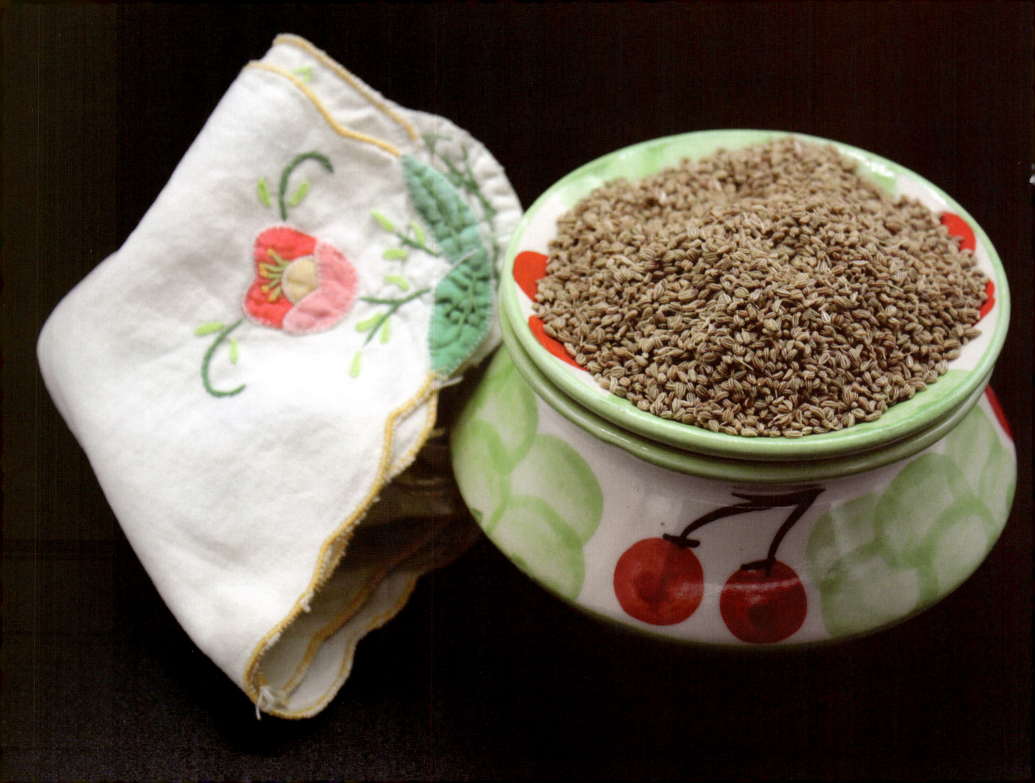

107. Ajmānō Śhēk (Carom Seeds Thermal Pack)
અજમાનો શેક

FOR RELIEF FROM WHEEZING, COUGHING, SORE THROAT

- Heat 2 tablespoons of **AJWAIN SEEDS** on a pan over very low heat and roast for 2-3 minutes

- Place the roasted seeds on top of a clean handkerchief and pack it together

- Test that the handkerchief hot pack is <u>hot enough on your skin without any discomfort or burning</u>. Then place it directly over the chest.

- Take 5-10 deep breaths to inhale the smell of the roasted seeds

- To maintain heat, press the pack on the heated pan for 5-10 seconds, test the pack on your skin and place over the chest

- Continue this process for 5-10 minutes

- Repeat 3 times a day as needed

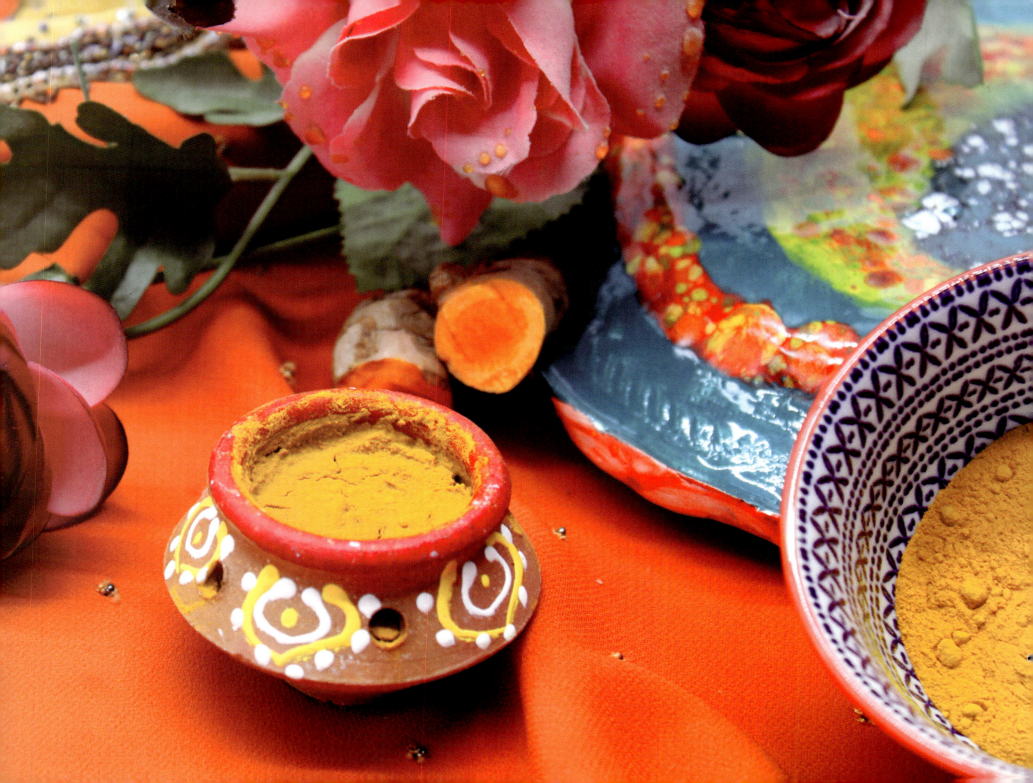

108. Haḍar Lagāvavī (Turmeric Topical Paste)
હળદર લગાવવી

FAST INJURY TREATMENT FOR CUTS AND WOUNDS

- Wash your hands

- Mix 1-2 teaspoons **ORGANIC TURMERIC POWDER** with enough **WATER** to form a thick paste. Alternatively mix 1-2 teaspoons of turmeric powder with ½ - 1 teaspoon of **PURE ORGANIC GHEE** to form a thick paste

- Gently apply the paste <u>on the wound</u>

- Cover with bandage wrap if desired

- Repeat after 12-24 hours as needed

Appendix A-D

*"No matter how much it gets abused, the body can restore balance.
The first rule is to stop interfering with nature."*
—Deepak Chopra

PREPARING YOUR MASALA BOX

Finding Indian spices is easier than you might think. Indian spices can be found at an Indian grocery store, health food store, supermarket, your garden or on the internet. Put spices of your choice in a traditional Masala Box (also known as _Masala Dabo_ - a container of spices). The Masala Box is an essential spice container rack that holds commonly used spices (masalas) in an Indian kitchen. The Masala Box is a round stainless steel container with seven small round tins that can hold & keep spices dry, small measuring teaspoon for spices and an inner lid that keeps the contents inside airtight and free from moisture.

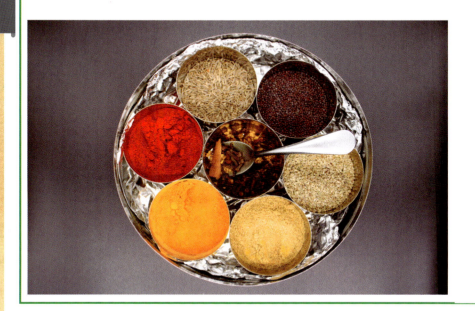
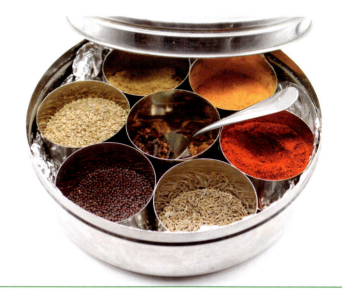

ESSENTIAL EQUIPMENT

BASIC

Assortment of Glasses (Glass, Copper, Stainless Steel)
Cups
Measuring Spoons
Measuring Glass
Tongs
Silverware (Spoon, Fork, Butterknife, Knife)
Stainless Steel Saucepan/Pot (Small and Large)
Mixing Bowl (Small and Large)
Coffee Grinder

SPECIAL

Mortar & Pestle (Granite, Stainless Steel, Wooden)
Masala Box (box of Spices)
Velan (Indian chapati wooden rolling pin)
Orasiyo (Indian round wooden chapati rolling board or marble slab)

RECOMMENDED RESOURCES

Support local grocers, Farmer's Markets and
other small business owners to buy Indian spices, herbs, and locally grown &
natural organic foods such as fresh fruits, vegetables, grains, seeds & nuts.

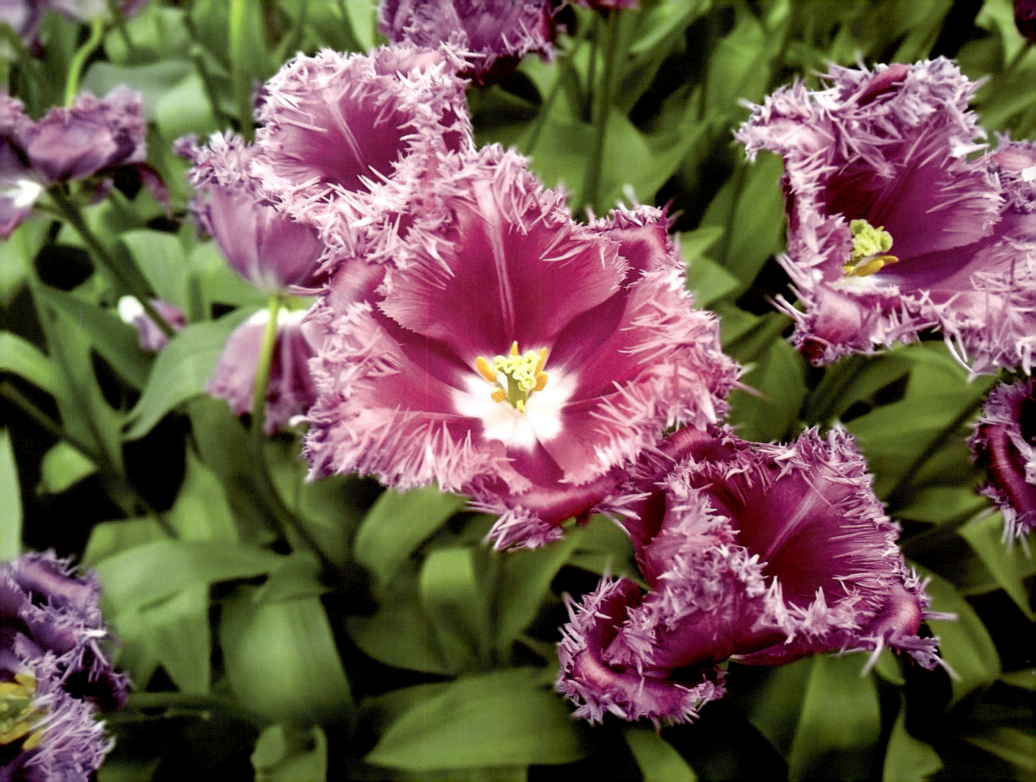

Significance of 108

"Samyak-Darśhan-Gyāñ-Chārītrānī-Mōkṣha-Mārgaha"

सम्यग्दर्शनज्ञानचारित्राणि मोक्षमार्ग

The right vision, right knowledge and right character (Ratnāṭrāẏā or triple gem of Jainism) *collectively constitutes the path to Moksha or liberation of karmic matter from the soul.*

—Tattvārtha Ādhīgām Sūtra by Acharya Umaswati, 2ⁿᵈ-5ᵗʰ Century AD

When I came to the United States in the 1970s there were not many Indians living here, much less Jain Indians. Growing up in New Jersey, we did not know many Jain families as not so many had emigrated from *India* yet. The medical doctors would tell my parents they needed to feed my brother and myself meat in order for us to grow and thrive. Much to the chagrin of the medical community and the society at large during the 1970s, I am thankful that my Mom and Dad were wise, held on to their roots and raised us as vegetarians. Growing up in New Jersey, I was exposed to many different religions at a young age and our family practiced the religion Jainism. A great portion of my life revolves around the religion, partly because my Father is a devoted Jain scholar/author and my Mother is also a published Jain author, but mostly because I am convinced of its core values. Namely, *Ahimsā* (non-violence), *Aparigrāha* (non-possessiveness) and *Anēkāntvāda* (non-absolutism, multiplicity of viewpoints, theory of relativity). The majority of my youth/adult life, cultural identity and personal ethics is centered around and informed by these principles. I apply them whenever possible. I feel fortunate to have been born into a Jain family and married into a Jain family as well. I am not intending to demean other religions and philosophies; just want to explain the spiritual value I've gained from Jainism. So you may be wondering, what is Jainism?

Jainism, one of the world's oldest religions, is different from Hinduism and Buddhism, and similarly originated from the Indian subcontinent. There are an estimated 10 million practitioners worldwide. Jainism is often classified as a way of living life with a rich philosophical and ethical system versus a religion by theologians. The word *Jain* is derived from the word "*Jina*" or conqueror/victor over the five senses. Jainism is a responsible, ethical and compassionate way of living and effectuates positive, nonviolent change in thought, action and deed. According to Jainism, the soul (*Atma* or life force) is weightless. As humans we do not have the power/strength to see our *Atma*. Jains believe that all living beings including animals, plants and microorganisms contain a soul or a life force. One of the main pillars of Jainism is compassion to all living beings. Jains believe each soul has equal value and every living being should be treated with compassion. According to science, every living being has a cell. The central tenet of Jainism is *Ahimsa* and this extends to not harming living beings physically (action), mentally (thoughts) and by speech (words). Jain philosophy promotes reverence for all forms of life and in the principles of peaceful co-existence of all living beings. Jainism is a way of life.

Jains follow a spiritually motivated vegetarian diet based on the principle of *Ahimsa* and one that minimizes harming any living organisms. We can practice *Ahimsa* in our interactions and try our best to not cause pain to any form of life including to our self (physical, mental, spiritual and emotional).

Important Jain practices around Ahimsa:

1. <u>No eating before sunrise and after sunset</u>. After sun down, temperature on earth decreases and this causes bacteria in the atmosphere to rapidly grow. Harmful microorganisms are in the air before the sun rises as well. To reduce risk of inadvertently killing innocent insects, injuring plants and eating food which has more microorganisms in the absence of sunlight, Jains don't eat after sunset and before sunrise.

2. <u>Drink boiled water daily</u>. After water is boiled, there are no living beings in the water and according to Jain thinking/science new life will not grow in that water for the next 9-15 hours. Jains boil water then filter and let it cool down before drinking it.

3. <u>No root vegetables, vegetarian diet</u>. Jains prevent injuring smallest of insects & microorganisms and excludes eating of root vegetables (ones that are grown in the soil such as potatoes, onions, garlic) as tiny life forms are injured and die when the plant is pulled up from the ground. As sunlight does not reach below the ground, each of these root vegetables contain infinite organisms living on it. Plucking those vegetables from the ground creates a sense of fear in those living organisms, destroys the entire plant and eating it would mean harming the living creatures (and countless souls) which is a type of violence. Jains do consume plants and fruits which are plucked above the ground as these are unicellular (one soul) and consumption of these plants & fruits involves minimum or least violence.

4. <u>No green, leafy vegetables on lunar hightide</u>. *Tithi* in Jainism translates to a "lunar day." This is calculated by the time it takes for the moon to increase its longitudinal angle from the sun by 12 degrees. Many vegetables have a water composition that is 90%+. Due to the lunar hightide on certain days of the month, it is believed that on those days the green leafy vegetables retain more water and therefore, growth of more living beings. To limit violence against these beings, Jains abstain from consuming green vegetables on the days of *Tithi* (half moon, full moon, etc). This practice of abstaining from consuming green vegetables on *Tithi* is a discipline over the attachment of the sense of taste. Our body has 80% water. Eating vegetables on the day of *Tithi* adds more water in our body. As a result the food does not digest easily.

Namōkār Mantra contains the essence of Jainism. This magical, all-powerful mantra (also known as *Navkar Mantra)* is the fundamental prayer in Jainism and can be recited by anyone (regardless of religion, caste or creed), at any time. This nine line *Mantra* does not refer to any specific God or saint. This universal prayer is a guide for attaining spiritual wealth. There are **108** <u>combined virtues</u> of five supreme spiritual beings which Jains worship when reciting this *Mantra.*

Namōkār Mantra

Namōkār Mantra	English Translation	Five Supreme Beings	Meaning of Five Supreme Spiritual Beings also known as *Panch Parmeshthi* in Gujarati Language	<u>108</u> Virtues
Ṇamō Arihantāṇaṁ	I bow down to *Arihantā* or *Tirthankara*	*ARIHANTA* or *TIRTHANKARA*	The souls who conquered inner enemies (attachment, anger, pride, greed) and have perfect knowledge of the past, present & future of the universe	12
Ṇamō Siddhāṇaṁ	I bow down to *Siddhā*	*SIDDHA*	The liberated souls who attained salvation by completely destroying all *Karma* (subtle, imperceptible karmic particles) and are free from the cycle of births & deaths	8
Ṇamō Ayariyāṇaṁ	I bow down to *Achārya*	*ACHARYA*	The spiritual leaders of the saints and congregation of monks, nuns, laymen & laywomen, and responsible for preservation of the noble path	36
Ṇamō Uvajjhāyāṇaṁ	I bow down to *Upādhyā*	*UPADHYAY*	The head teacher saints of the scriptures and dissemination of their knowledge of the philosophical systems to the monks, nuns, laymen and laywomen	25
Ṇamō Lōē Savva Sāhūṇaṁ	I bow down to *Sādhu* and *Sādhvi*	*SADHU* and *SADHVI*	The saints in the universe who have renounced from worldly aspects of life for spiritual upliftment – all *Sadhu* (Monks) & *Sādhvi* (Nuns)	27
Ēsō Pañcha Ṇamōkkārō	My bowing downs represent physical & mental salutations towards these five most esteemed, supreme spiritual beings,			
Savva Pāva Paṇāsaṇō	will diminish and destroy all sins and obstacles,			
Maṅgalā Ṇaṁ Cha Savvēsiṁ	and amongst all the auspicious mantras,			
Paḍamam Havaī Maṅgalaṁ	this *Namokar Mantra* is the first & foremost. May the virtues of these five supreme beings guide & inspire me to progress spiritually through the Jain code of conduct (right faith, right knowledge, right conduct) and achieve the ultimate goal of total liberation from the bondages of *Karma* also known as *Moksha* (or *Nirvana*).			

The *Jain Mālā*, or garlands of *Mantra* prayer beads, come as a string of 108 beads, which signify the 108 attributes (or combined virtues) of these five supreme spiritual beings. Jains believe that *Karma* is a physical substance (subtle, invisible, microscopically imperceptible karmic particles) that pervades everywhere in the entire universe and karmic matter is attracted to the soul by actions of that individual soul. Karma in Jainism is a natural universal law and all souls - men & women - have the potential to attain *Moksha* (liberation). According to Jainism, there are 108 number of ways (by activities of mind, speech and body) with which the influx of new karmic particles can be attracted to the soul. The ultimate goal is liberation from the bondages of *Karma* which are constantly attached to the soul.

The numbers 9, 12 and 108 have spiritual significance in many cultures, religions, traditions and philosophies.

- $9 \times 12 = 108$
- $1 + 0 + 8 = 9$

- 108 is a Harshad number, a positive integer that is divisible by the sum of its digits (108 is divisible by 9)

- $1^1 \times 2^2 \times 3^3$ ($1 \times 4 \times 27$) $= 108$

- The inner angles in degrees formed by two adjacent lines in a regular pentagon equals 108 degrees

- The average distance of the Sun to Earth, and the average distance of the Moon to Earth is 108 times their respective diameters.

- 108 degrees Fahrenheit is the internal temperature at which the human body's vital organs begin to fail from overheating

108 *is a magical, mystical and powerful number in Jainism*
and connects humanity & the world —
ancient, modern, future.

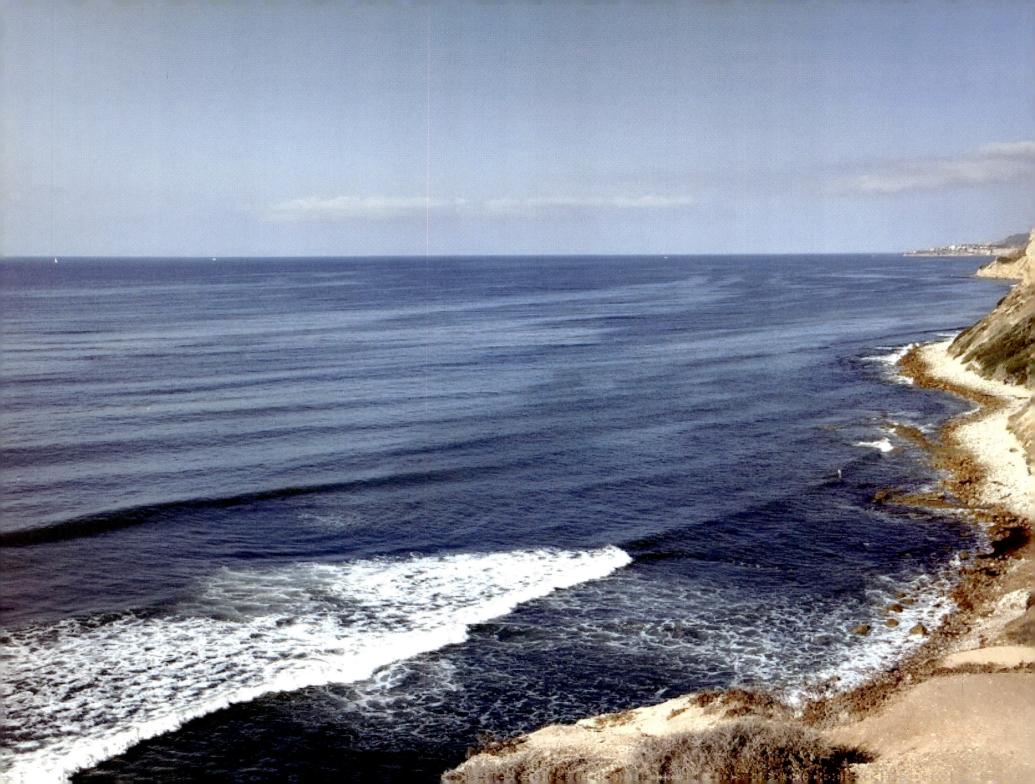

12 Lifestyle Practices

*"Don't accumulate if you do not need. The excess of wealth in your hands
is for the society, and you are the trustee for the same."*
—Mahāvīra Bhaghwān

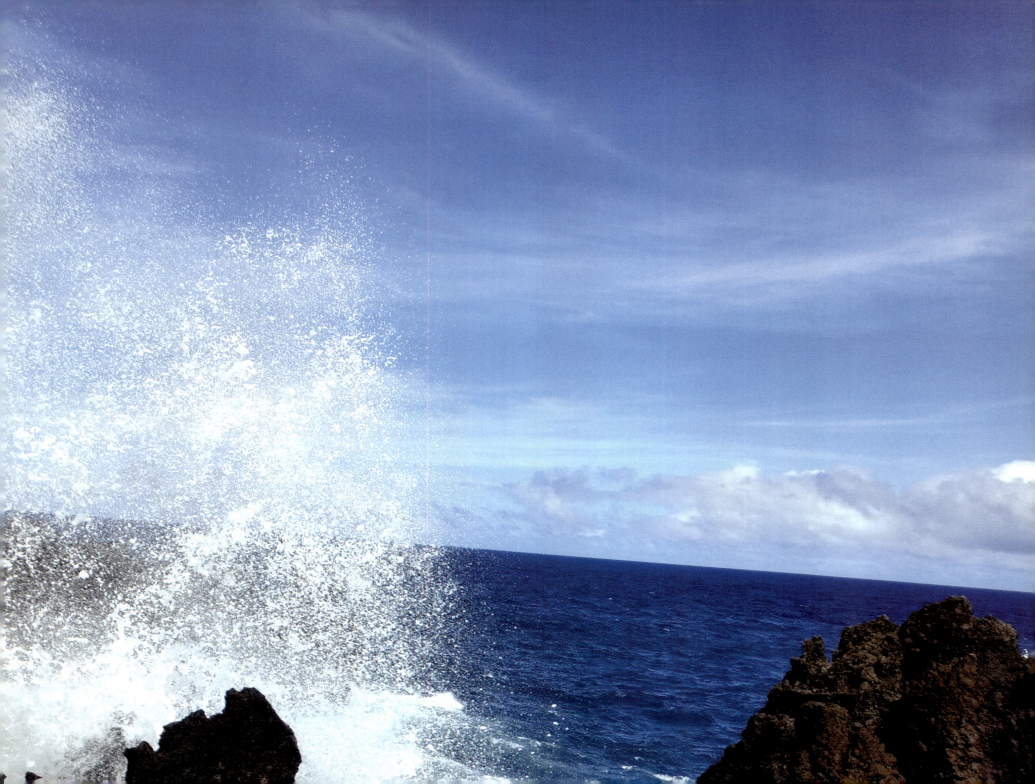

I. Ukāḷēlu Pāṇī (Drink Boiled Water)

ઉકાળેલુ પાણી

FOR GENERAL HEALTH

- In the early morning add approximately 1 gallon of tap **WATER** to a large deep pot

- When bubbles start to form, the boiling process has begun. Wait for a few minutes to let bubbles come to a rolling boil for a total of 3 times According to Jainism and the Centers for Disease Control and Prevention (CDC), boiling water kills disease-causing organisms including viruses, bacteria, germs, protozoans and parasites

- Pour this purified water into a large deep dish (or multiple deep dishes) and let it cool

- Filter the water through a clean cloth or coffee filter, then transfer to a clean sanitized container and cover with a lid

- Enjoy this purified, filtered water for drinking throughout the day

    Do not put this water in the refrigerator

    Do not add any other water or salt in this water

    According to Jainism this water is safe to drink for next 9-15 hours

    Drink this water <u>between sunrise and sunset</u> and throw out the water after dusk

- Repeat daily

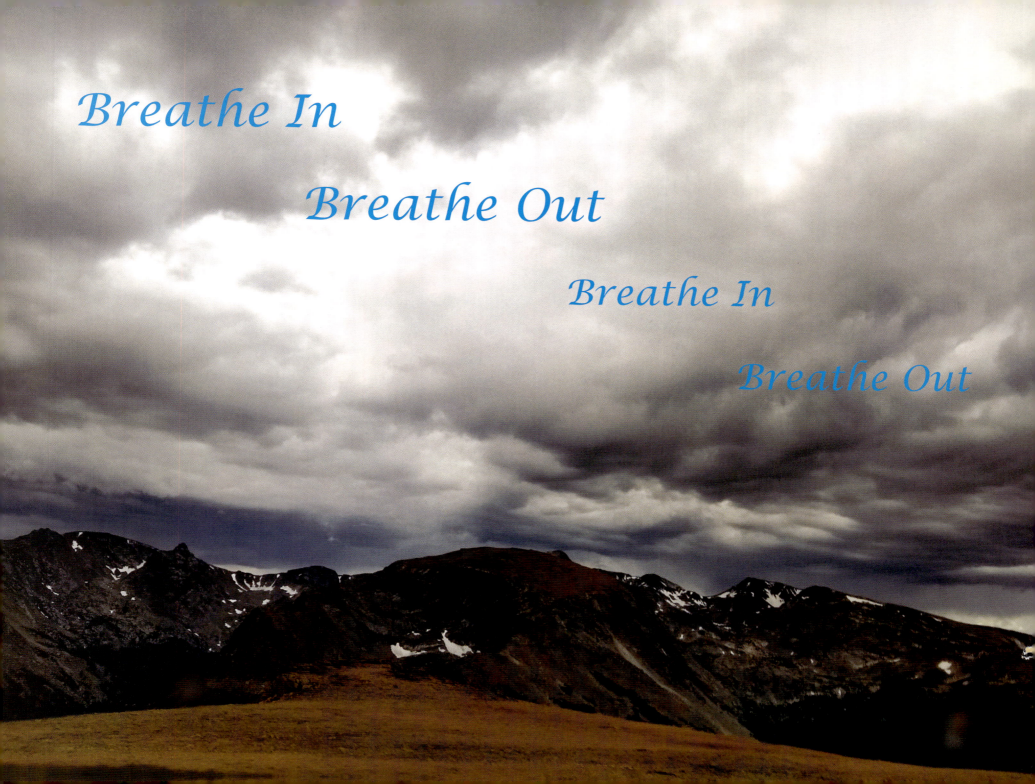

II. Lāmbā Svāśh Lēvā (Deep Breathing Meditation)
લાંબા શ્વાસ લેવા

FOR GENERAL HEALTH & DETOXIFICATION, DECREASE STRESS, RELAX THE MIND

- Find a comfortable, quiet place that you can relax. Sit with your head, neck and back straight on the floor, in a chair, on a sofa. You decide. Or you can be in a standing posture. Close your eyes

- Take **DEEP BREATHS**
  - Slowly Breathe In: during your inhale, observe your breath going, invite in positive thoughts
  - Pause: hold it in as long as your are comfortable
  - Slowly Exhale Out: during the exhale, observe your breath going out, release negativity and stress

- Take another deep inhalation
  - Become aware of your breath again. Pay attention to the air entering and exiting from your nose
  - Become a silent observer and use your breath as an anchor, watching the thoughts come and go
  - Slowly recite the beautiful and powerful OM mantra

- Continue this for 5-10 minutes (or as long as you are comfortable)

- When you're ready gently open your eyes

- Repeat mindful breathing meditation practice (schedule time on your calendar to start 1x/week and slowly ramp up to a daily practice)

Do You
slow down and
CHEW
your food?

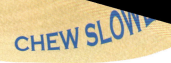

III. Dhīmēthī Chāvvānu (Chew Slowly)

ધીમેથી ચાવવાનું

FOR EFFICIENT DIGESTIVE SYSTEM AND BETTER FOOD & NUTRIENT ABSORPTION

- Sit down to eat each of your meals in a day (leave your technology devices in another room)

- With each bite of food, chew your food **32 TIMES** thoroughly and slowly with your mouth closed

- After the *food* has lost all texture and turned into a complete liquid, you can swallow slowly

- Now rest to savor the taste of food and take a refreshing breath

- Pick up the next bite to eat and chew 32 times per mouthful before swallowing

- Repeat this mindful eating practice for each morsel of food you eat and remember to rest in between bites & chew your food more slowly

- Wait at least 30 minutes after each meal to drink water

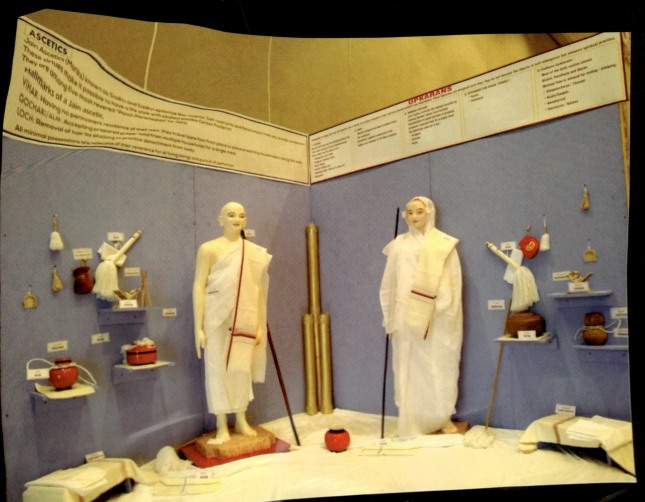

A Daily Practice

Get UP & Move

IV. Rōj Chālvānu Rākhō (Walk Daily)

રોજ ચાલવાનું રાખો

FOR GENERAL HEALTH

- **WALK** continuously for 1 hour at your preferred speed (preferably outdoors)

- Make this *simple* <u>lifestyle change</u> and repeat daily

- Go on a walking meditation where you are aware of each step. Jain Monks and Nuns (*Sādhu-Sādhvī*) walk for 10-12 hours a day. They walk carefully to avoid stepping on insects and not injure living creatures

- Whether you are fit or unfit, make a practice to get up and move around for 5 minutes every 30 minutes during the day

- Take walking 1:1s versus office meetings. Walking meetings can increase creativity, inspire new ideas, enhance relationship building and improve your life and health

- Shut down your phone, turn off social media and walk away from the laptop. Go meet with your family members and friends in a casual stroll

- Stand when reading emails and stand/walk when you are talking on the phone

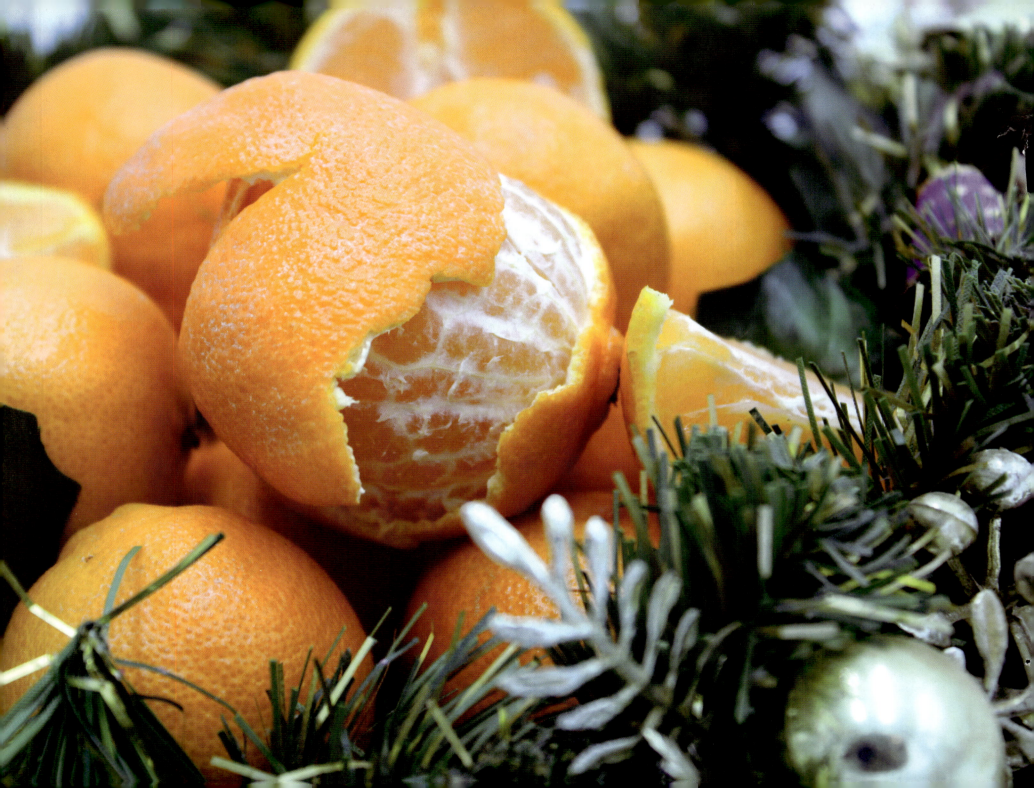

V. Sāttvik Bhōjan Khāvānu (Eat Fresh, Ethical, Natural)

સાત્ત્વિક ભોજન ખાવાનું

FOR GENERAL HEALTH, PEACEFUL MIND

- Eat locally grown **SIMPLE, PURE, HEALTHY, VEGETARIAN/PLANT-BASED/VEGAN MEALS** every day in moderation

- Have your meals sitting on the floor in a cross-legged position (known as *Sukhasana* in yoga), bend forward to take a bite *&* return back to natural posture to chew and swallow your food

- Sattvik foods are nourishing vegetarian foods that brings mind into balance & keeps the body in harmony. This includes fruits, nuts, legumes, seeds, ghee, oil, whole grains, vegetables, organic dairy

- Follow Jain vegetarian/Jain vegan motivated diet that exemplifies the doctrine of *Ahimsa*

  Minimize harm to other living organisms

  Avoid eating roots and tuber vegetables/plants grown underground such as potatoes, onion, garlic

  Do not eat meat, seafood, poultry, eggs, mushroom, fungus, yeast. Do not drink beer, wine, alcohol

- Avoid consumption of packaged, canned & processed foods, and food stored overnight

- Enjoy nutritious, sattvic meals with love *&* gratitude for a well-rounded eating practice (moderate sized breakfast, large lunch and small dinner <u>with no food wastage</u>)

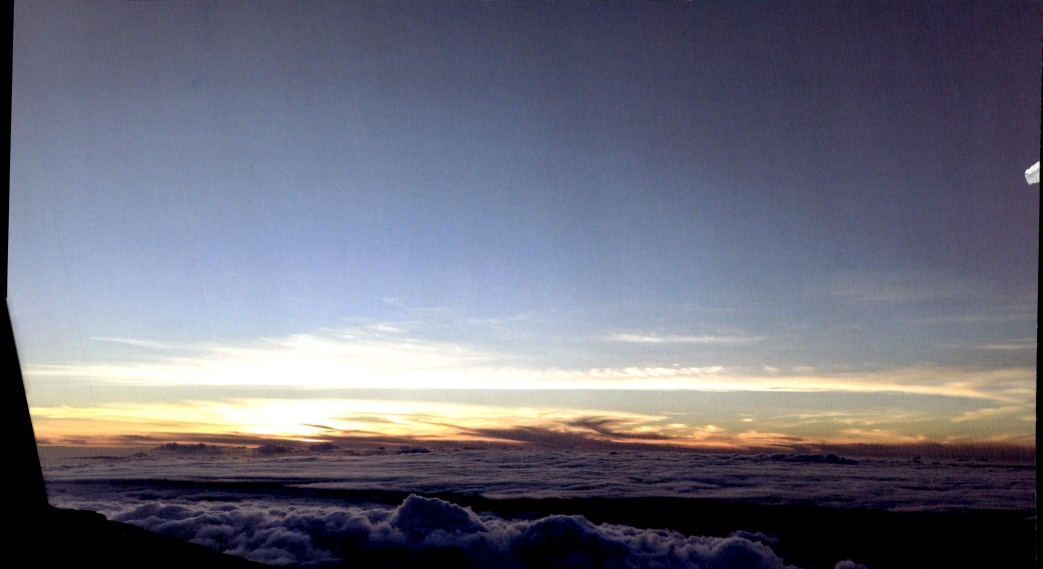

VI. Śhānti Thī Suvānu (Sleep Well)

શાંતિથી સુવાનું

FOR GENERAL HEALTH

- Have **SOUND SLEEP** every night
- Strive for consistent early sleeping/waking times (early to bed, early to rise)
- <u>Two hours before going to bed:</u>
    Avoid eating and drinking fluids
    Stop using electronic devices (TVs, smartphones, laptops, monitors, tablets…)
    Turn off bright lights
- Go to the bathroom before going to bed
- In bed, sleep on left side (or tilting your head on left side) and practice meditation. Close your eyes and focus on one thing
- Think about what you are grateful for from the day
- When you wake up in the morning, close your eyes and take a few moments to reflect on what you are grateful for in your life
- Take a deep inhale and slowly recite OM mantra out loud or internally
- Repeat powerful mantra total 108 times to invoke positive energy inside you

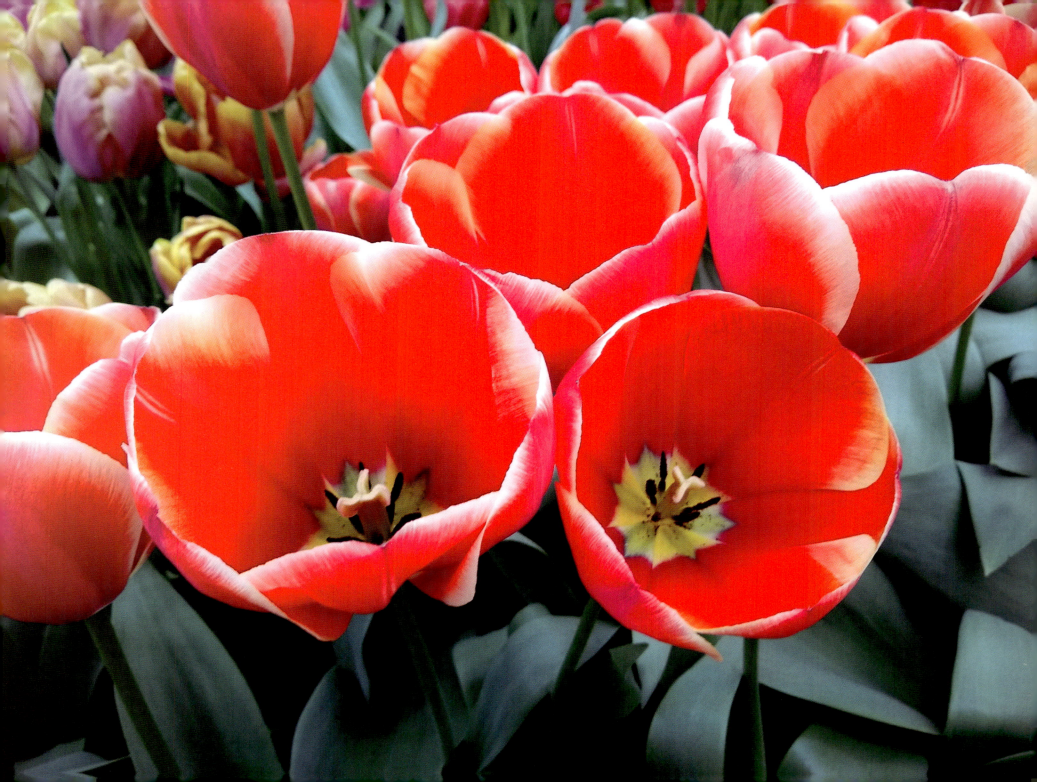

VII. Sārā Vichār Karvānā (How to Positively Think)

સારા વિચાર કરવાના

FOR GENERAL HEALTH

- Embrace the power of **POSITIVE THINKING** in all aspects of life each day. Smile more and laugh more

- Live intentionally with a positive outlook and watch your energy shift

- Suspend judgment (don't judge). <u>Look for the positive qualities</u> in others and take time to appreciate the small things in life

- Be fully present, engaged and aware of where you are in the present moment

- Read good books to learn, inspire & adopt a positive mental attitude, unlearn negative thinking and change your thoughts for the better

- Develop a daily practice of gratefulness. Take a few moments each day to reflect on what you are grateful for in your life

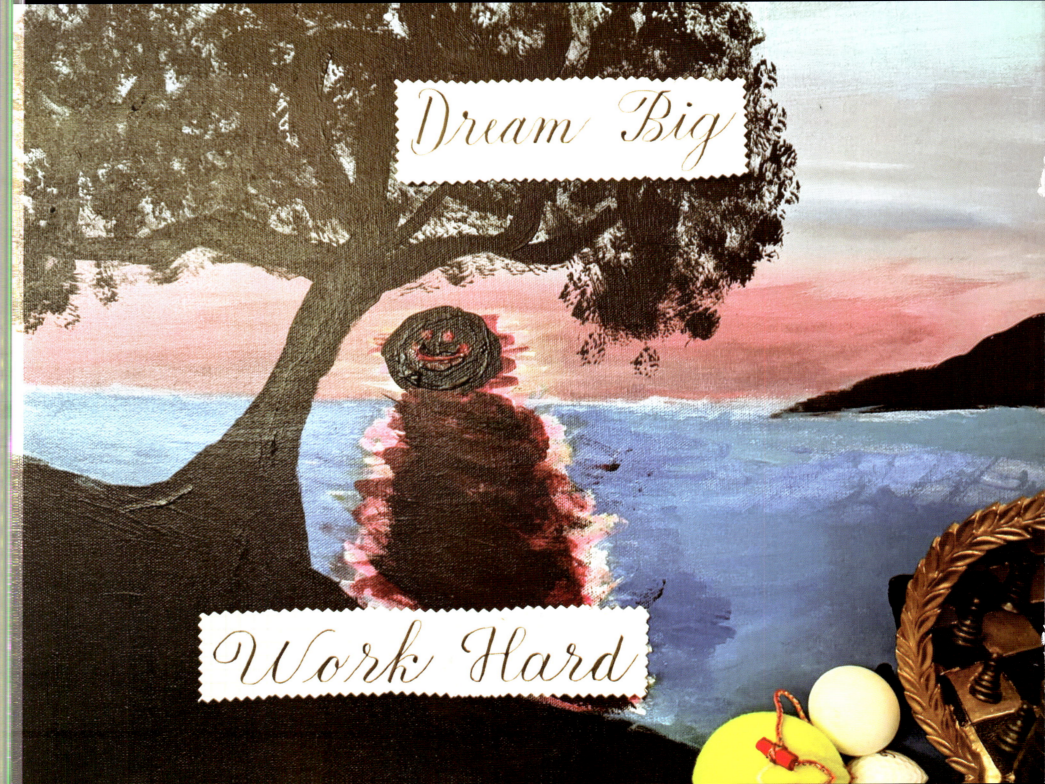

VIII. Mahēnat Kārō (Work Hard)

મહેનત કરો

TO ACHIEVE GOALS

- Write down **GOALS** for your career and personal life

- Add key milestones and assign those to your timeline. For example, an overarching goal may be to get more fit in next 9 months and milestones can include getting a membership to the local gym, beginning a fitness routine and then reducing processed foods

- Developing the discipline to think and plan increases the odds of a successful outcome

- Dedicate time to focus on your area (read, study, practice)

- Work on improving your core strengths by scheduling time each day to exercise core muscles, eat more fruits/vegetables and eliminate processed foods from your diet. You'll feel stronger and sharper which will improve your productivity at work and at home

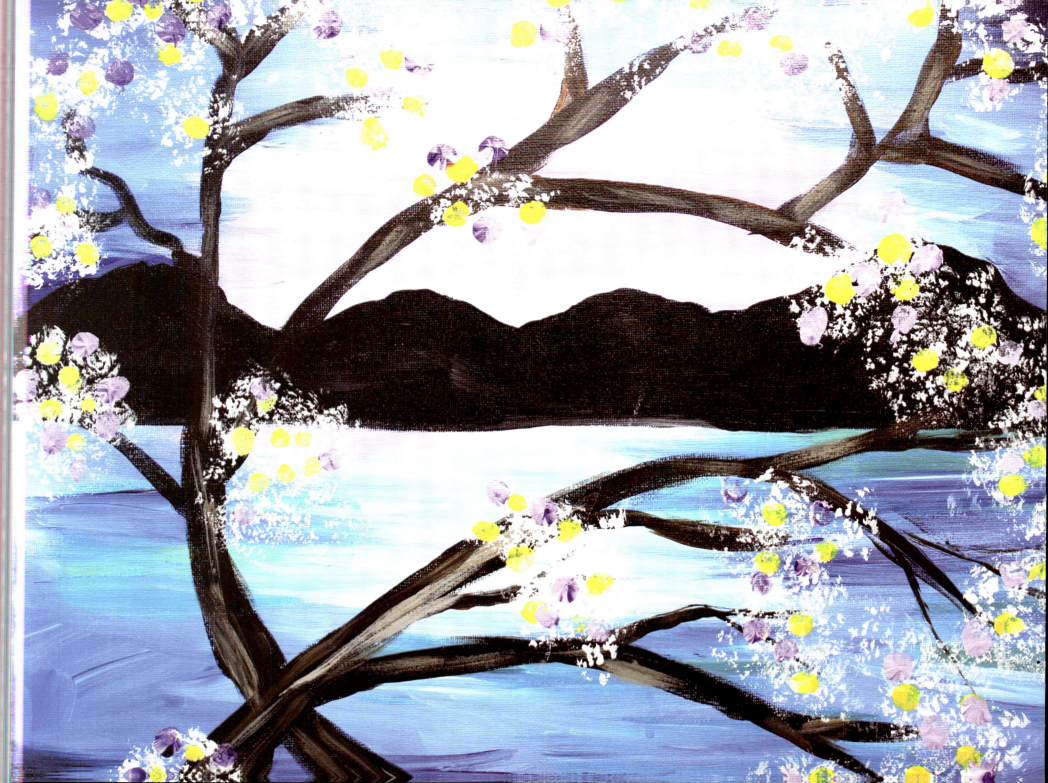

IX. Apēkśhā Rākhvānī Nahī (Live Without Expectations)

અપેક્ષા રાખવાની નહી

THE KEY FOR HAPPINESS

- <u>Lower</u> your **EXPECTATION(S)** from
  - ➢ Family
  - ➢ Relatives
  - ➢ Friends

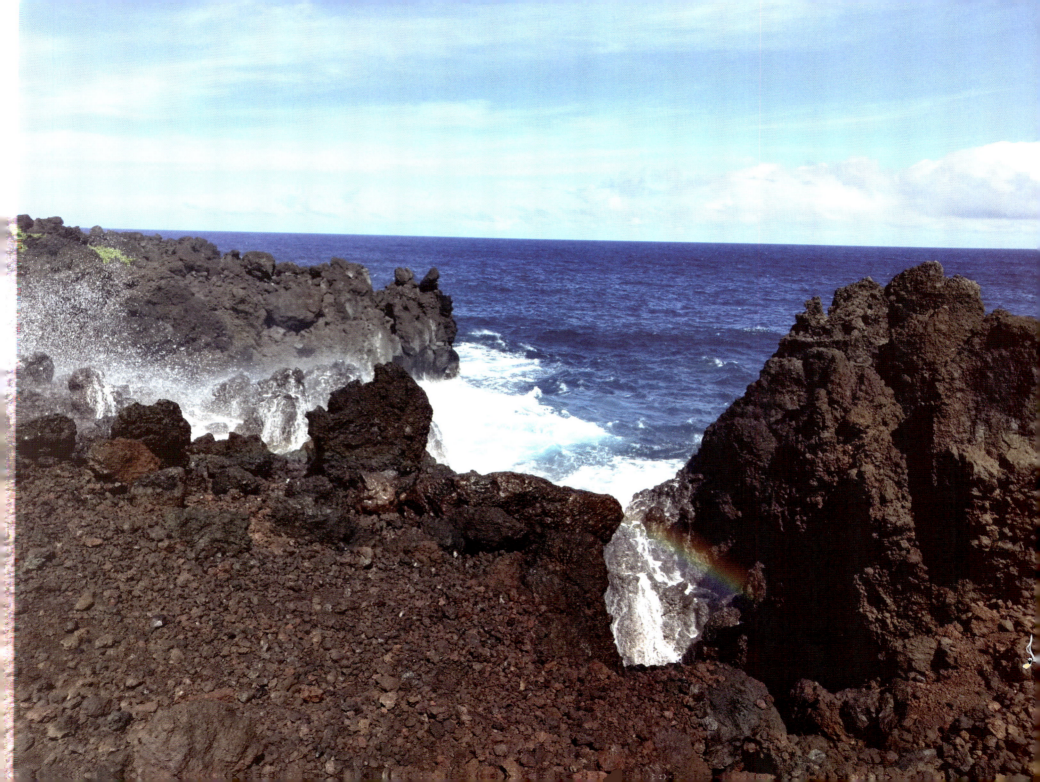

X. Dhīraj Rākhō (Learn to Wait)

ધીરજ રાખો

TAKE CONTROL OF YOUR MENTAL REMOTE CONTROL & LEARN TO PAUSE

- Make an effort to <u>be in charge of your thoughts, feelings & reactions</u> rather than jumping to conclusions, going on auto-pilot and reacting in ways that we sometimes regret

- When faced with differences/conflicts:

  - Control your emotions

  - Focus on your breathing

  - Pause to let the mind settle

  - Recite OM to self-manage, relax the mind and calm the body

  - **WAIT 24 HOURS** before reacting and before responding (in person, verbally, via email, on social media, etc)

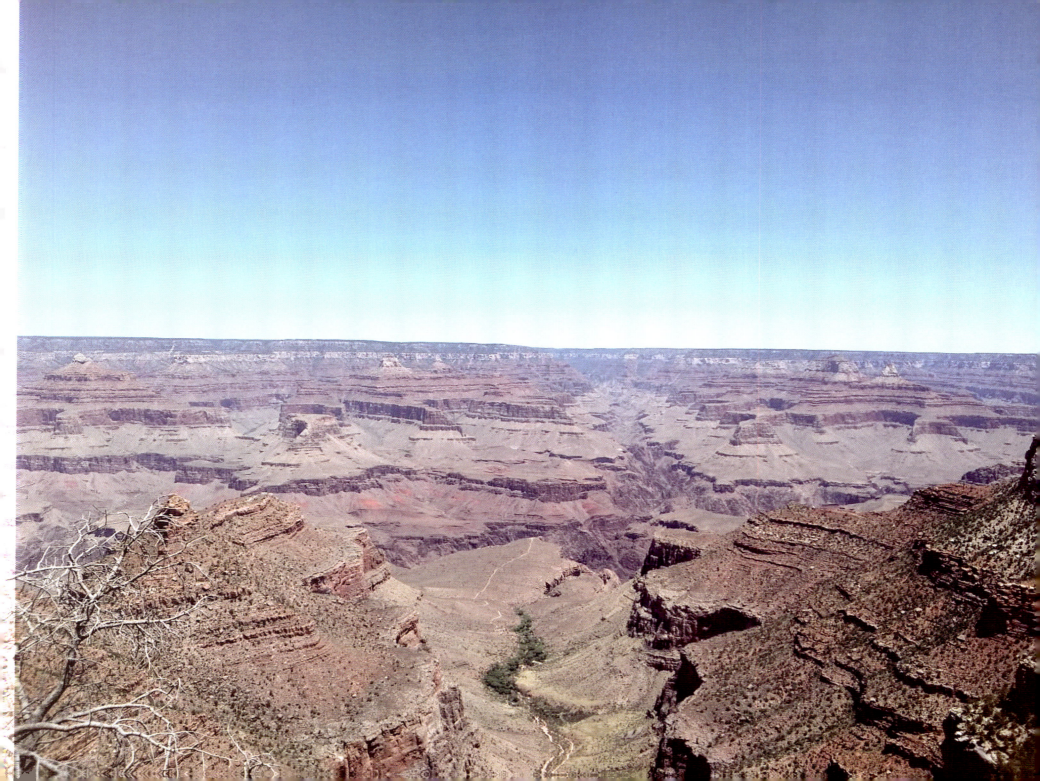

XI. Madhyastha Rahēvānu (Remain Centered)
મધ્યસ્થ રહેવાનું

TO STAND IN THE MIDDLE, STAY CENTERED

- Make a **CONSCIENTIOUS** effort to stop having attachment (*Rag*) and hatred (*Dwesh*) on anyone or anything. Have friendship towards all and animosity towards no one

- Overcome desire for revenge by controlling your emotions, showing compassion and reaching out for forgiveness If you are deprived of what you like or want, do not react with anger (*Krodh*). If someone breaks your trust or does something against what you wished for, don't let the mighty anger flare up. Anger leads to seeking revenge which could involve some level of mental violence

- When critical feedback is given to you, don't listen to the voice of the ego (*Mana*) and do not let ego take control of you. Push the ego aside, stay tranquil and truly listen. If you do not get credit/recognition/spotlight for your effort and accomplishments, drop the ego and focus your mind on self-satisfaction for a job well done

- Be honest. Deceit (*Maya*), deception, lying and dishonesty are acts of manipulation, destroys trust and are rooted by low self-esteem. Develop courage and tell the truth

- Be content with what you have, have a generous spirit and give back to the world at large. Greed (*Lobh*) is an immunity to satisfaction. Avoid the temptation of excess and wanting more, e.g. power, wealth, food, possessions/things

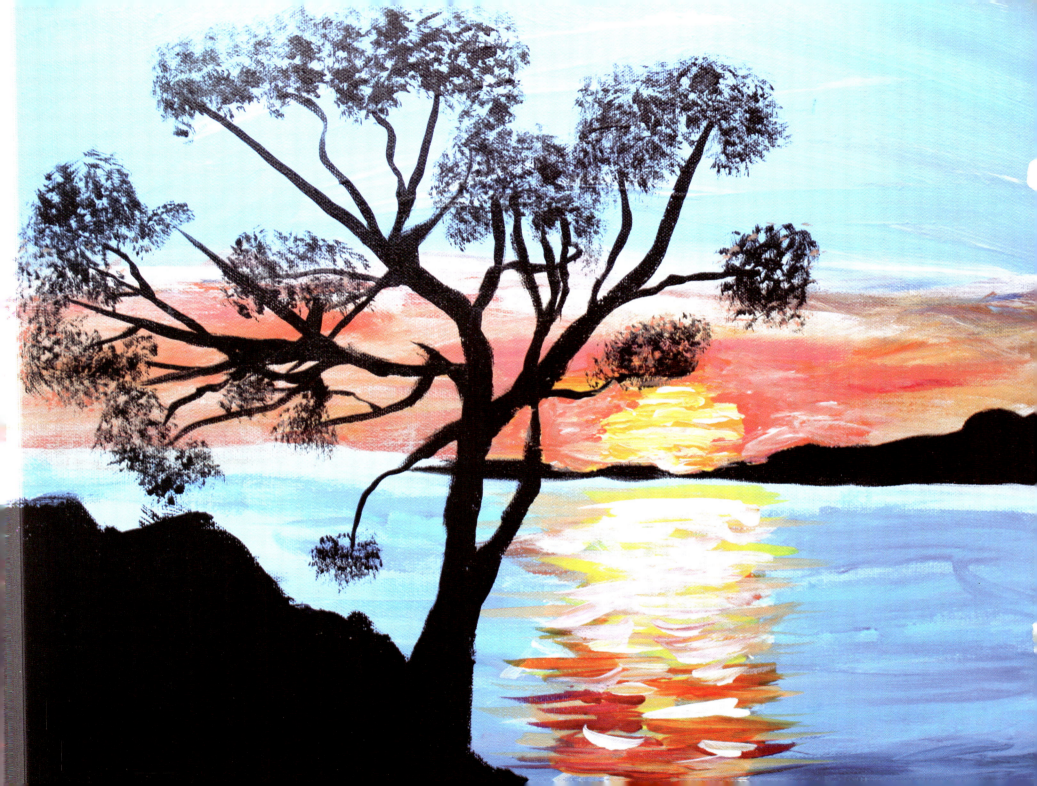

XII. Sūrya Kālē Paṇ Ugaśhē (Sun Will Rise Tomorrow)

સૂર્ય કાલે પણ ઉગશે

To Hope

- The sun **WILL RISE** tomorrow
  - Muster the strength
  - Rise and stand tall
  - Keep hope alive
  - Don't let your thoughts control you
  - Move forward
- Trust that <u>this moment will pass</u> and it gets better

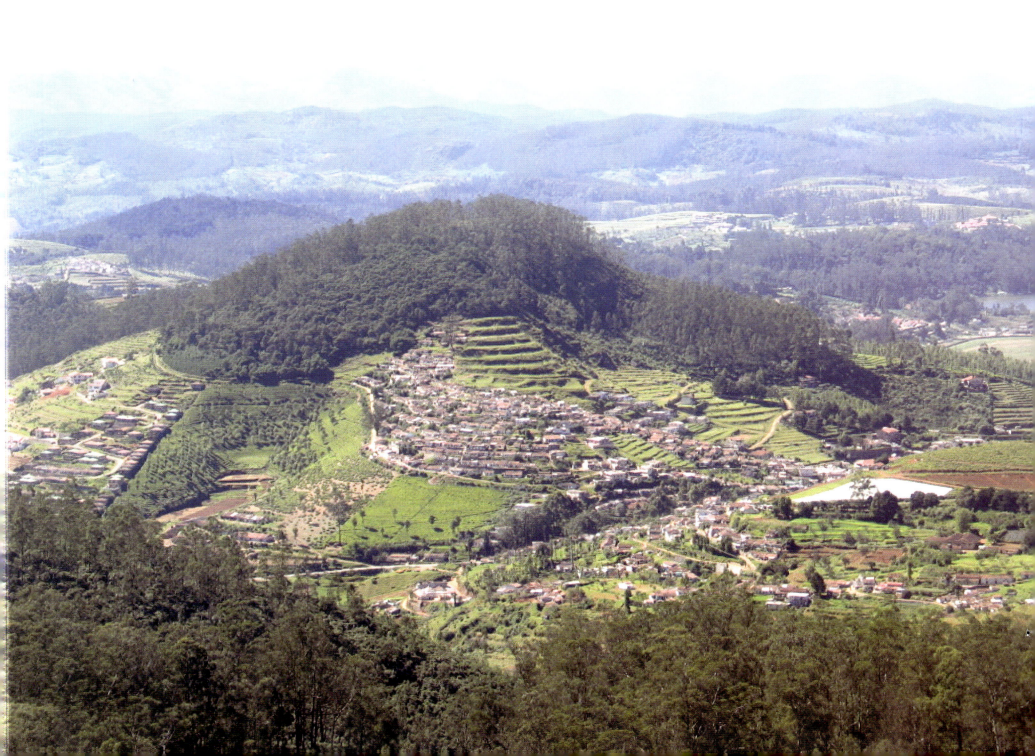

Glossary of Ingredients

"Hard work never brings fatigue. It brings satisfaction.
Once we decide we have to do something, we can go miles ahead."
—Prime Minister Narendra Modi

English	Gujarati	Medicinal Benefits*	I	G	W
Ajwain	Ajmo	Digestive aid. Good for indigestion, stomach pain. Relieves headache, cough, cold. Smoke of seed acts as bronchodilator. Controls cholesterol	✓		✓
Almonds	Badam	Anti-oxidant. Lowers LDL-cholesterol levels, blood pressure. Reduces heart disease. Rich source of vitamins and minerals. Help trigger weight loss.	✓	✓	✓
Amla (Indian Gooseberry)	Amla	Anti-oxidant. Lowers total cholesterol and triglyceride levels. Anticarcinogenic. High in fiber and vitamin C. Protects the brain. Builds immunity. Manage blood sugar levels.	✓		✓
Asafoetida	Hing	Anti-spasmodic, anti-inflammatory. Aids digestion. Treats indigestion, IBS, flatulence, bloating. Digestive aid. Relieves asthma, cough, menstrual pain	✓		✓
Cardamom	Elaichi	Anti-oxidant, Antimicrobial, Anti-carcinogenic, diuretic. Improves nausea, gas, acidity. Good for gastrointestinal health, cardiovascular health.	✓		✓
Castor Oil	Deevel	Relieves muscle/joint pain. Natural laxative. Moisturizes skin. Promotes healing of wounds. Reduces acne. Conditions hair.	✓		✓
Chana Dal	Dalia	Good source of fiber, protein. Reduces inflammation. Lowers cholesterol. Aids digestion. Improves constipation and as a snack for weight loss.	✓		✓
Chili	Marchu	Anti-inflammatory. Digestive relief from gas, stomach pain, cramps. Aids in circulation, excessive blood clotting, high cholesterol, hangover.	✓	✓	✓
Cinnamon	Taj	Anti-oxidant. Anti-inflammatory. Anti-spasmodic. Normalizes blood sugar levels. Fights bacterial infections. Reduces heart disease risk factors.	✓	✓	✓
Clarified Butter	Ghee	Anti-inflammatory. Rich in vitamins A, D, E & K. Shelf stable. High in monosaturated Omega-3S. Moisturizes dry skin and hair.	✓	✓	✓
Clove	Laving	Anti-oxidant. Anti-inflammatory. Anti-carcinogenic. Anti-viral. Improves motion sickness. Increases metabolism. Digestive aid. Topical analgesic.	✓	✓	✓
Copper	Tamba	Drinking water from copper vessel is great brain stimulant. Regulates functioning of thyroid gland. Aids in weight loss. Boosts digestive health.	✓		✓
Copper Zinc Tin	Kansa	Copper improves joint pain, inflammation. Zinc boosts immune system. Improves digestive system performance. Relieves headache and insomnia.	✓		✓

Availability   I - Indian Store   G - Local/National Grocer   W - Online Retailer

English	Gujarati	Medicinal Benefits*	I	G	W
Coriander	Dhanajeeru	Anti-inflammatory. Anti-spasmodic. Rich in calcium, vitamin C, iron. Useful for bone pain. Lowers cholesterol. Digestive aid.	✓		✓
Cumin	Jeeru	Anti-carcinogenic. Promotes digestion, sleep. Rich in iron, potassium. Improves morning sickness, indigestion. Muscle relaxant.	✓	✓	✓
Edible Gum Crystals	Goondh	Strengthen immune system, stamina, health. Rich in protein, calcium, iron. Aids in constipation. Prevents heat strokes.	✓		✓
Eucalyptus Oil	Nilgiri	Soothes sore muscles. Eases muscle tension, swelling		✓	✓
Fennel	Variyali	Breath freshener. Promotes sleep. Reduces stress. Helpful for indigestion, bloating. Improves eyesight. Relieves joint pain. Regulates blood pressure.	✓		✓
Fenugreek	Methi	Rich in protein, vitamins A, C, iron, calcium, minerals. Lowers cholesterol. Stimulates milk production in nursing mothers. Improves digestion.	✓		✓
Fig	Anjeer	Anti-oxidants. Powerhouse of fiber. Rich in vitamins A, C, K, B, potassium, magnesium. Alleviates constipation. Aids digestion. Natural laxative.		✓	✓
Fuller's Earth	Multani Mati	Improves blood circulation. Unclogs skin pores. Treats acne. Improves skin elasticity, glow. Fades scars. Prevents split ends. Relieves tired limbs.	✓	✓	✓
Ginger	Aadu	Anti-inflammatory, anti-viral, anti-bacterial, anti-carcinogenic Relieves joint pain, cold, flu, headaches, arthritis pain, fevers, GI irritation, nausea.	✓	✓	✓
Gram Flour	Besan	Rich source of fiber, vitamins and minerals. Lowers cholesterol levels. Controls diabetes. Healthy alternative to gluten. Helps treat acne. Improves heart health. Prevents fatigue.	✓	✓	✓
Haritaki	Harde	Anti-aging properties, relieves constipation. Beneficial for weight loss, stomach related problems, mouth ulcers.	✓		✓
Honey	Madh	Anti-oxidant. Lowers blood pressure, LDL cholesterol & triglyceride levels. Promotes topical wound healing. Suppresses cough.	✓	✓	✓
Jaggery	Gol	Anti-allergic. Detoxifies body Immune boosting. Rich in iron and fiber. Blood purifier. Prevent joints pain and constipation. Digestive agent.	✓	✓	✓

Availability   I - Indian Store   G - Local/National Grocer   W - Online Retailer

English	Gujarati	Medicinal Benefits*	I	G	W
Millet Flour	Bajri	Relief from cough and cold.	✓	✓	✓
Moong Beans	Moong	Antioxidant, anti-inflammatory, anti-microbial. Packed with potassium, protein, fiber, magnesium, phytonutrients, vitamins A, C. Heart healthy.	✓		✓
Mustard Seeds	Rai	Anti-inflammatory, anti-bacterial. Lowers blood pressure. Rich in A, B-complex, C vitamins, magnesium. Provides relief from cold, sinus.	✓		✓
Nutmeg	Jaifal	Anti-oxidant, anti-inflammatory, anti-septic. Treats anxiety, depression, insomnia, bleeding gums, toothache. Aides digestion. Improves memory.	✓	✓	✓
Papadum	Papad	Aids digestion. High in protein, dietary fiber. Enhances taste of an Indian meal (note: this is high in sodium so consume in moderation).	✓		✓
Peepramul	Pipramul	Aids digestion, appetite. Relieves gas, bloating, heartburn, constipation, asthma, joint pain. Treats stomach ache, menstrual cramps.	✓		✓
Poppy Seeds	Tal	Anti-oxidant defense. Improves digestion. Calming effect on the brain, induces sleep. Increases energy levels. Strengthens bones, connective tissue.	✓		✓
Saffron	Kesar	Anti-oxidant. Anti-inflammatory. Improves visual acuity. Protection against glaucoma. Helpful for macular degeneration. Relieves depression. Treats PMS symptoms.	✓	✓	✓
Sandalwood	Chandan	Improves focus, concentration, positive energy. Relief from headache.	✓		✓
Tongue Scraper	Uliu	Removes bacteria. Reduces bad breath. Improves tongue's appearance, sense of taste. Boosts immune function. Promotes general tooth/gum health.	✓		✓
Triphala	Trifala	Improves vision. Eye rejuvenation, revitalization. Good for general eye care.	✓		✓
Turmeric	Haldar	Anti-oxidant, anti-inflammatory, anti-septic, anti-carcinogenic, anti-bacterial, anti-allergic. Immune boosting. Reduces pain, inflammation. Digestive healing agent. High in curcumin. Mango Turmeric (known as "Amba Haldar" in Gujarati) has similar benefits as turmeric.	✓	✓	✓
Walnut	Akhrot	Anti-oxidant. Heart healthy. Good for brain health and hair. Reduces risk of cancer.	✓	✓	✓

Availability   I - Indian Store   G - Local/National Grocer   W - Online Retailer

Glossary of Terms

*"You have to find what sparks a light in you
so that you in your own way can illuminate the world."*
—Oprah Winfrey

Teaspoon	Tablespoon	Fluid Oz	Cup
48 tsp	16 Tbsp	8 oz	1 cup
36 tsp	12 Tbsp	6 oz	¾ cup
32 tsp	11 Tbsp	5 oz	⅔ cup
24 tsp	8 Tbsp	4 oz	½ cup
16 tsp	5 Tbsp	3 oz	⅓ cup
12 tsp	4 Tbsp	2 oz	¼ cup
6 tsp	2 Tbsp	1 oz	⅛ cup
3 tsp	1 Tbsp	½ oz	¹⁄₁₆ cup

dash	medium sized lemon	2 cups	4 cups, 2 pints	16 cups 8 pints 4 quarts
~⅛ tsp	2-3 Tbsp juice	1 pint	1 quart	1 gallon

½ inch Peeled Turmeric Root = 1 teaspoon Turmeric Powder

Sources/ References

"Happiness is when what you think, what you say, and what you do are in harmony."
—Mahatma Gandhi

Sources

Preface
- whc.unesco.org/en/list/1551 - United Nations Educational, Scientific and Cultural Organization

Glossary of Ingredients and Glossary of Terms
- webmd.com - online news and information pertaining to health and well-being
- healthline.com - online health guidance
- en.wikipedia.org - online encyclopedia
- medicalnewstoday.com - web-based outlet for medical news
- food.ndtv.com - online source for food news, health news, Indian recipes
- chopra.com - provider of experiences, and education for the well-being of body, mind and spirit
- whfoods.com - not for profit foundation to eat and cook for healthy health
- livestrong.com - nonprofit org that provides support for people affected by cancer
- tarladalal.com - India's best-selling cookery author
- thehealthsite.com - online health guide
- foodfacts.mercola.com - online site on food and nutrition
- dictionary.com - online dictionary

Significance of 108
- studyjainism.org - online site to learn the basics of Jain religion
- ancientpages.com/2017/06/19/ - secret and powerful number 108 that has accompanied mankind

Lifestyle Practices (1. Ukāḷēlu Pāṇī – Drink Boiled Water)
- cdc.gov - Centers for Disease Control and Prevention

References
- *Tattvartha Adhigam Sutra* by Chandrakant B. Mehta - philosophical text on Jainism on path of liberation
- *Amari Navvanu Yatra no Mitho Anubhav* by Pravina C. Mehta - experiences during 99 day pilgrimage
- JAINA.org - nonprofit federation of Jain Association in North America

INDEX

"Life's most persistent and urgent question is: What are you doing for others?"
—Dr. Martin Luther King, Jr.

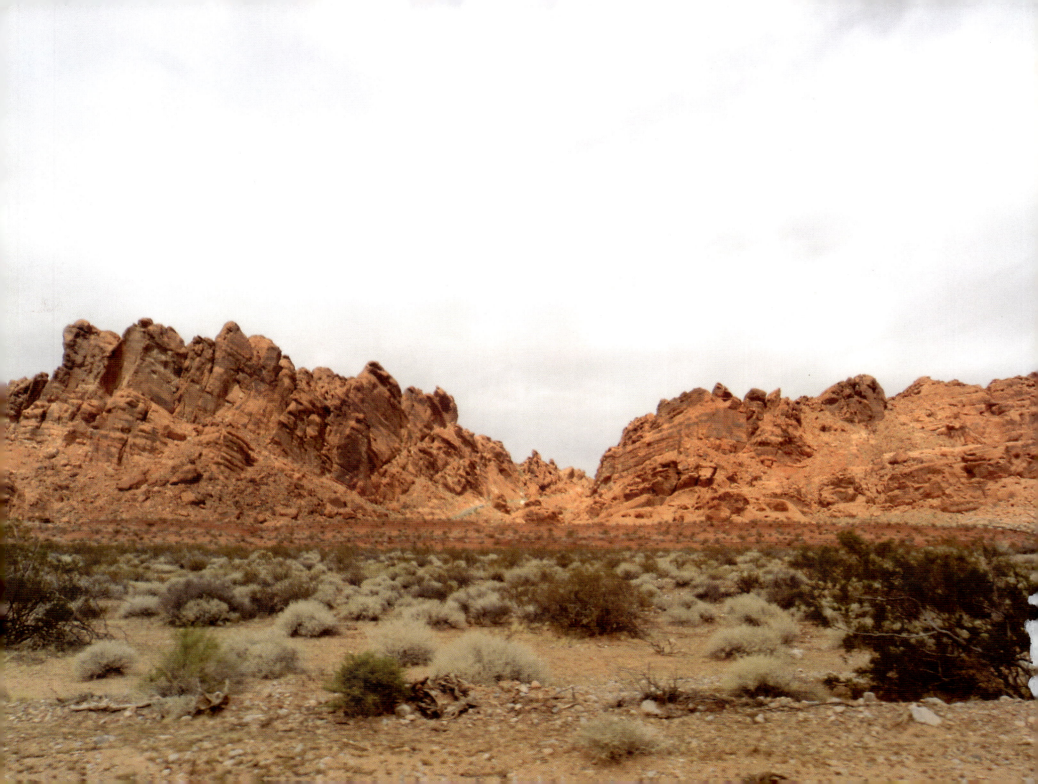

Gratitude

"Every living being has a strong desire to live and we must respect this in our thoughts and actions."
—*Mahāvīra Bhaghwān*

...To my dear Family!

Mommy, you are the most organized, disciplined, hard-working and beautiful woman (inside & out) that I have met in my life. None of this would have happened without your support, wealth of knowledge & edits of many, many draft copies over 18 months. Thank you from the bottom of my heart.

Daddy, you are my role model. Thank you for pouring your heart into every page and helping bring it to life. I appreciate the granularity and thought from correcting Gujarati, Jainism & Practices sections to grammar of the remedies. I learned a lot on entire book publishing process with your experiences in authoring several books.

Saavan & Sunay, you are pillars for Pappa and me. We are blessed to have the most wonderful children a parent could ask for. Our gifts to you both: roots of a treasured past and wings with the freedom to fly & soar. Thank you for believing in my vision for this book. You helped me see the light when I wanted to put it back on the shelf... so many times! I appreciate your help to choose the perfect words, thoughtful commentary on the book/pics & format/edits of various sections over 18 months. You inspire me daily to reach for the stars.

Sujal, I am the luckiest woman in the world. I appreciate your faith in me to use home remedies for so many years and your support in my initiative to write the book & create photo studios throughout our home! Your honest, invaluable feedback on the content/photos inspired me to improve and build my confidence. Thank you for supporting my dreams in every way possible with your uniquely brilliant eye.

Manish, thank you for being my brother. Appreciate you taking the time to read and critique early drafts & one of the final versions of the book. Your comments sharpened the work and gave me encouragement to think differently about the next steps.

Dillan & Amani, you are the coolest nephew & niece. SujalFua and I are proud of your accomplishments. Your reviews of the book and feedback on the photographs & content have been helpful. Thanks!

Family & Friends, you know who you are. It took over 18 months from having a first draft copy for editorial review to getting this book published. You shared advice on home remedies to me & my family at some point during the past five decades and/or helped me get this book across the finish line to first print by providing valuable suggestions, technical assistance, content review or photography feedback.

I appreciate you all very much. Thank you for giving me so much of you, your time, love & support.

I am very thankful to both Bharatbhai and Jineshbhai (Bharat Graphics Ahmedabad) for their beautiful typesetting, timely printing, and valuable suggestions. Khub Khub Anumodana.

Lastly my humble Pranam to all extended family members who are partners with Sujal, Sunay, Saavan & me in this lifetime.

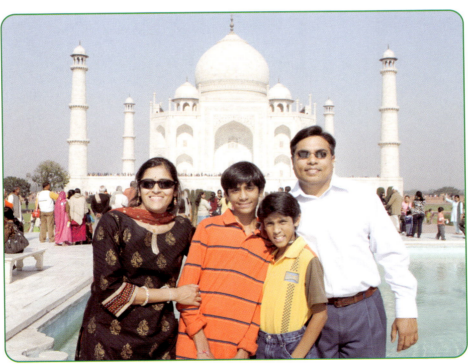

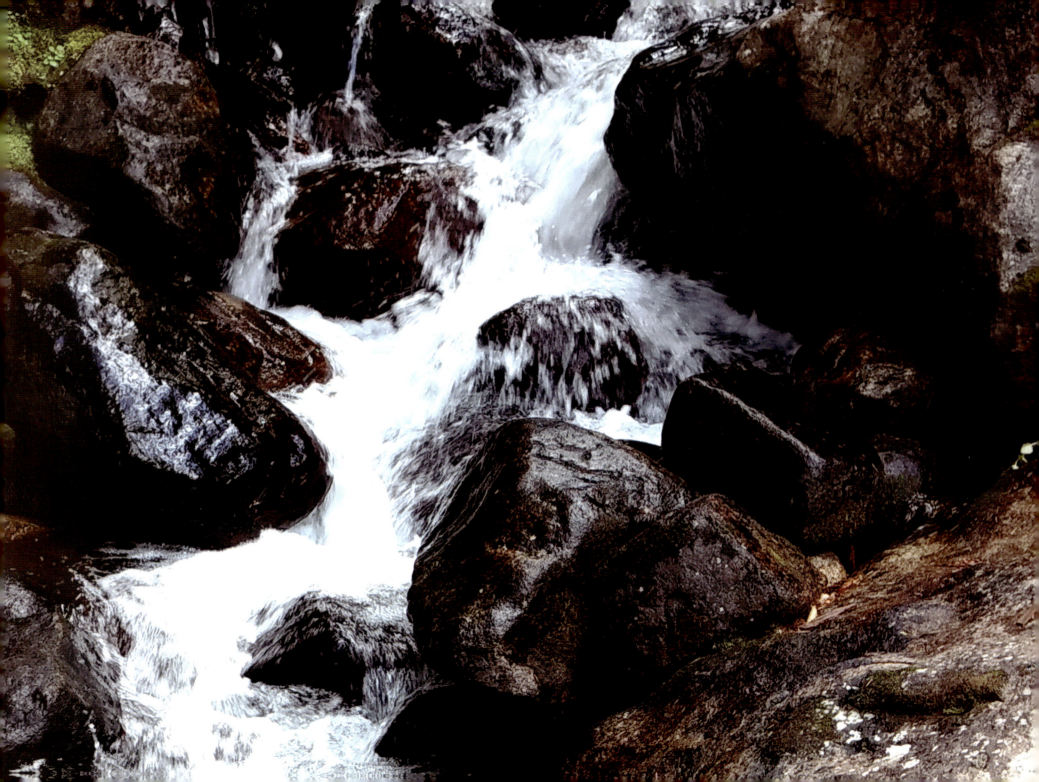

Author's Note

*"This is our time… And where we are met with cynicism and doubts and those who tell us that we can't, we will respond with that timeless creed that sums up the spirit of a people: **Yes, we can**."*
—President Barack Obama, Victory Speech 2008

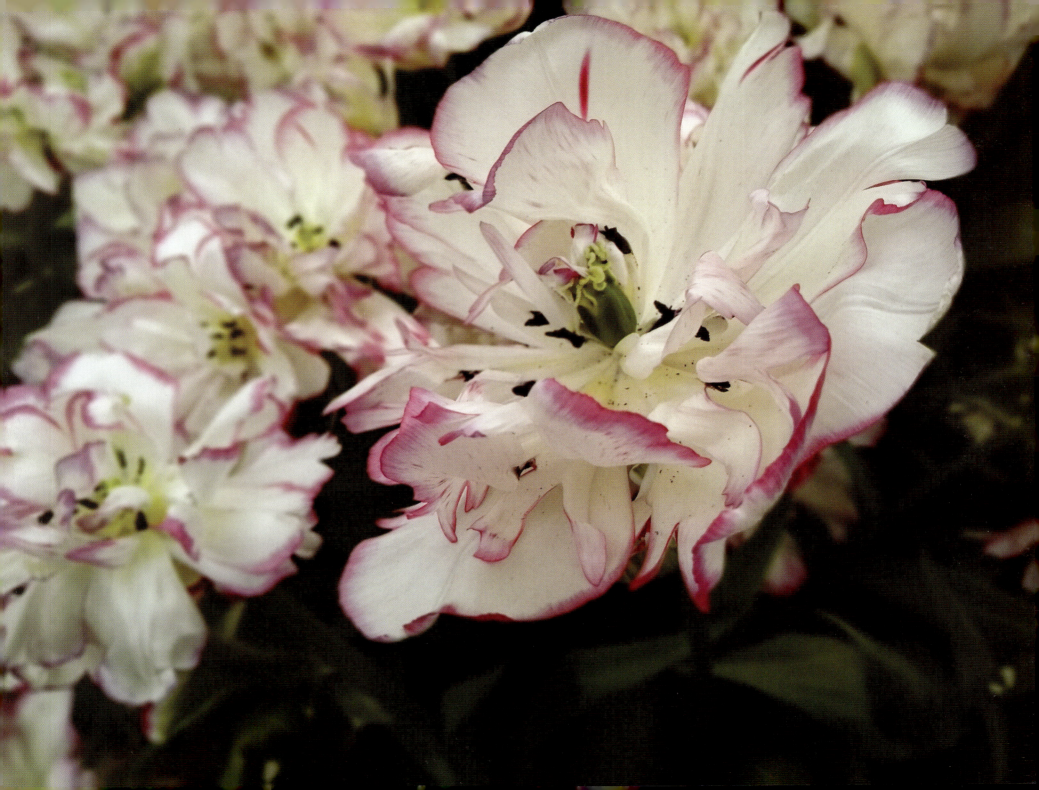

This book is not meant to be read cover to cover.

Flip to a page that interests you and read it twice ("measure twice, cut once").

Feel free to follow the steps in the remedy for best results.

Next time you have a need or interest, flip to a page that interests you and read it twice...

Repeat as needed.

You can now close the book.

Thank you!
Binny Sujal Nanavati

ps - If you found this book helpful, consider dropping
a brief review on Amazon or retailer of your choice, & tell a friend.

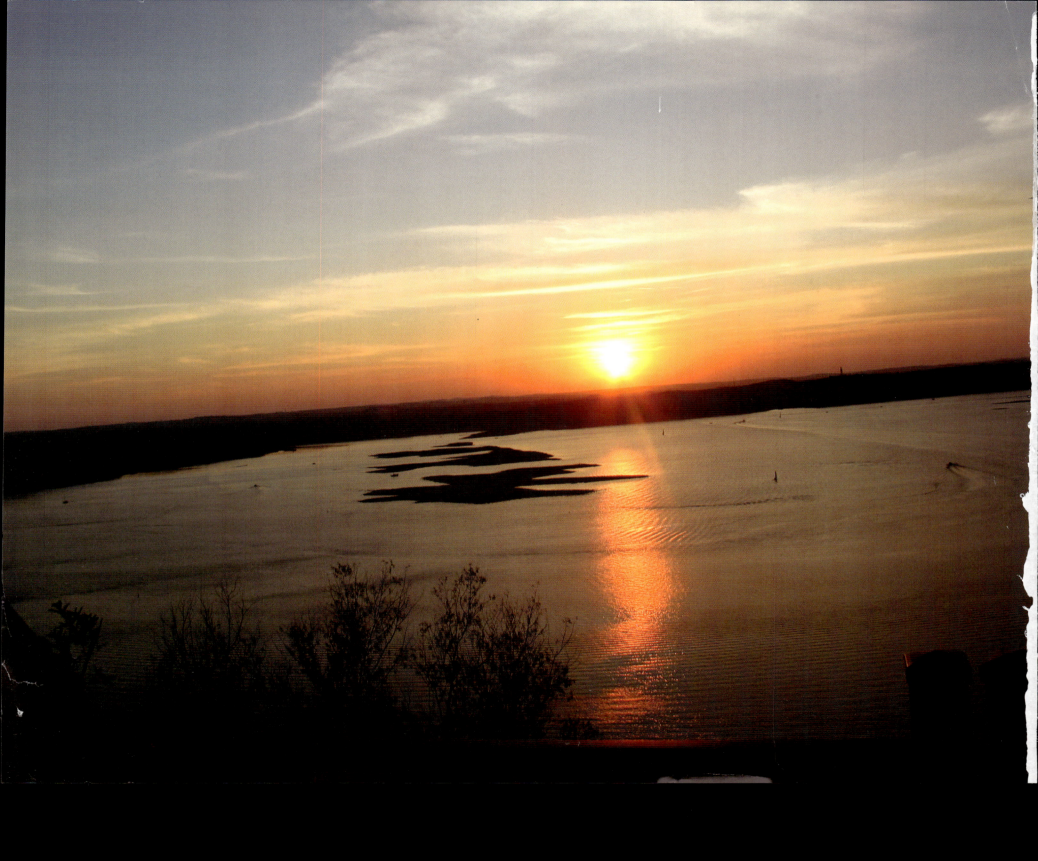

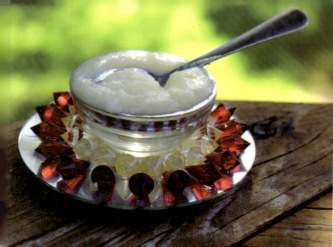
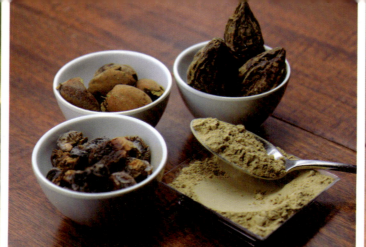
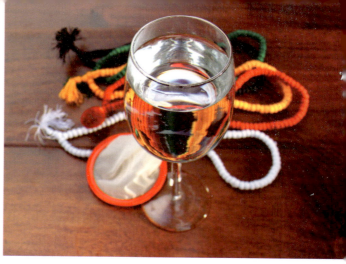
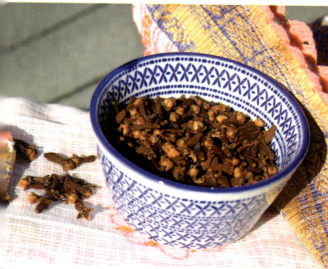

108

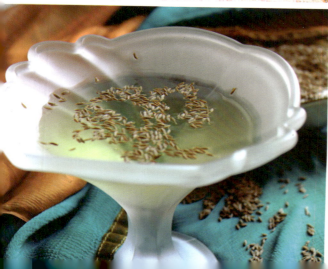
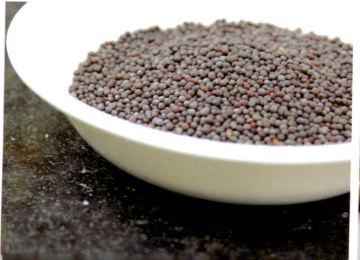
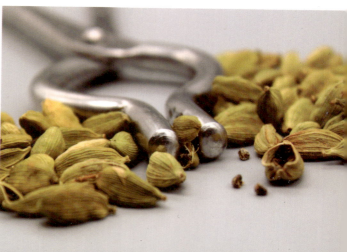